W9-AEV-043

DISCARDED

ANNUAL REVIEW OF NURSING RESEARCH

Volume 9, 1991

EDITORS

Joyce J. Fitzpatrick, Ph.D.
Dean and Elizabeth Brooks Ford
  Professor
Frances Payne Bolton School of
  Nursing
Case Western Reserve University
Cleveland, Ohio

Ada K. Jacox, Ph.D.
Professor and Independence
  Foundation Chair
The Johns Hopkins University
School of Nursing
Baltimore, Maryland

Roma Lee Taunton, Ph.D.
Associate Professor
School of Nursing
University of Kansas Medical Center
Kansas City, Kansas

Associate Editor

Nikki S. Polis, Ph.D.
Researcher
Frances Payne Bolton School of
  Nursing
Case Western Reserve University
Cleveland, Ohio

ADVISORY BOARD

Jeanne Quint Benoliel, D.N.Sc.
Professor Emeritus, School of
  Nursing
University of Washington
Seattle, Washington

Doris Bloch, Dr.P.H.
National Center for Nursing Research
National Institutes of Health
Bethesda, Maryland

Ellen O. Fuller, Ph.D.
School of Nursing
University of Pennsylvania
Philadelphia, Pennsylvania

Susan R. Gortner, Ph.D.
School of Nursing
University of California, San
  Francisco
San Francisco, California

Ada Sue Hinshaw, Ph.D.
National Center for Nursing Research
National Institutes of Health
Bethesda, Maryland

Janelle C. Krueger, Ph.D.
College of Nursing
Arizona State University
Tempe, Arizona

Angela Barron McBride, Ph.D.
School of Nursing
Indiana University
Indianapolis, Indiana

Joanne Sabol Stevenson, Ph.D.
College of Nursing
The Ohio State University
Columbus, Ohio

Harriet H. Werley, Ph.D.
School of Nursing
University of Wisconsin—Milwaukee
Milwaukee, Wisconsin
Founding Editor
Annual Review of Nursing Research

Margaret A. Williams, Ph.D.
School of Nursing
University of Wisconsin—Madison
Madison, Wisconsin

ANNUAL REVIEW OF NURSING RESEARCH

Volume 9

Joyce J. Fitzpatrick, Ph.D.
Roma Lee Taunton, Ph.D.
Ada K. Jacox, Ph.D.

Editors

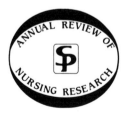

SPRINGER PUBLISHING COMPANY
New York

CARL A. RUDISILL LIBRARY
LENOIR-RHYNE COLLEGE

RT
81.5
.A55
v9
154417
Dec.1991

Order ANNUAL REVIEW OF NURSING RESEARCH, Volume 10, 1992, prior to publication and receive a 10% discount. An order coupon can be found at the back of this volume.

Copyright © 1991 by Springer Publishing Company, Inc.
All rights reserved

No part of this publication may be reproduced, stored in a retrieval system, or transmitted in any form or by any means, electronic, mechanical, photocopying, recording, or otherwise, without the prior permission of Springer Publishing Company, Inc.

Springer Publishing Company, Inc.
536 Broadway
New York, NY 10012

91 92 93 94 95 / 5 4 3 2 1

ISBN-0-8261-4358-X
ISSN-0739-6686

ANNUAL REVIEW OF NURSING RESEARCH is indexed in *Cumulative Index to Nursing and Allied Health Literature and Index Medicus.*

Printed in the United States of America

Contents

PREFACE

The *Annual Review of Nursing Research* series has been a significant addition to the scientific literature in nursing. Research reviewed for Volume 9 follows the established format for five major parts: Nursing Practice, Nursing Care Delivery, Nursing Education, the Profession of Nursing, and Other Research. Authors are selected based on their research expertise in an identified area. In their review and analysis of the literature, authors have contributed to the development of nursing knowledge for the discipline. They also have continued to project future research directions. These critical reviews and future projections set the stage for continued discipline growth.

The chapters under Nursing Practice for the present volume are primarily focused on human responses to chronic illness. Vickie A. Lambert reviews research on arthritis, Meridean Maas and Kathleen Buckwalter review research on Alzheimer's disease; Shirley A. Murphy examines human responses to catastrophe; Barbara A. and Charles W. Given analyze research on family caregiving for the elderly; and Joan K. Austin evaluates research on family adaptation to a child's illness. Chapters in this area in Volumes One and Four were focused on human development along the life span, chapters in Volume Two on family, and Volume Three on community, Volume Five on human responses to actual and potential health problems, chapters in Volume Six on specific nursing interventions, and chapters in Volume Seven and Eight on physiological aspects of nursing.

In the area of nursing care delivery, Pauline Komnenich and Carolyn Feller examine disaster nursing research and Mattilou Catchpole reviews research on nurse anesthesia care. In the section on nursing education, as in previous volumes, there is a focus on areas of specialized clinical education. Bonnie Rogers reviews research on occupational health nursing education. Research on the profession of nursing includes a chapter by Connie Vance and Roberta Olson on mentorship.

In the area of other research, two chapters are included. Noni L. Bodkin and Barbara C. Hansen review nutritional studies in nursing and Margaret A. Newman reviews health conceptualizations. In this section we are interested particularly in including international nursing research; we have targeted chapters in future volumes that will be focused on nursing research in other countries. We welcome your suggestions for authors from other countries to review the nursing research in that country.

The success of the *Annual Review* series has been enhanced by the contributions of the distinguished Advisory Board. We thank them for their suggestions and appreciate their advice and support. We also acknowledge the critiques of anonymous reviewers and the editorial and clerical assistance provided by support staff at Case Western Reserve University, the University of Kansas, and the Johns Hopkins University.

As always, we welcome readers' comments and suggestions for shaping the upcoming volumes. Please let us know your interests in contributing potential chapters to the series and your comments on this volume.

JOYCE J. FITZPATRICK
SENIOR EDITOR
ARNR SERIES

Contributors

Joan K. Austin, D.N.S.
Indiana University
School of Nursing
Indianapolis, Indiana

Noni L. Bodkin, Ph.D.
School of Medicine
University of Maryland-Baltimore
Baltimore, Maryland

Kathleen C. Buckwalter, Ph.D.
College of Nursing
University of Iowa
Iowa City, Iowa

Mattilou Catchpole, Ph.D.
School of Health and Human Services
Sangamon State University
Springfield, Illinois

Carolyn Feller, Ph.D.
College of Nursing
Arizona State University
Tempe, Arizona

Barbara A. Given, Ph.D.
College of Nursing
Michigan State University
East Lansing, Michigan

Charles W. Given, Ph.D.
College of Human Medicine
Michigan State University
East Lansing, Michigan

Barbara C. Hansen, Ph.D.
School of Medicine
University of Maryland-Baltimore
Baltimore, Maryland

Pauline Komnenich, Ph.D.
College of Nursing
Arizona State University
Tempe, Arizona

Vickie A. Lambert, D.N.Sc.
School of Nursing
Medical College of Georgia
Augusta, Georgia

Meridean L. Maas, Ph.D.
College of Nursing
University of Iowa
Iowa City, Iowa

Shirley A. Murphy, Ph.D.
School of Nursing
University of Washington
Seattle, Washington

Margaret A. Newman, Ph.D.
School of Nursing
University of Minnesota
Minneapolis, Minnesota

Roberta K. Olson, Ph.D.
School of Nursing
University of Kansas Medical Center
Kansas City, Kansas

Bonnie Rogers, Dr.P.H.
School of Public Health
University of North Carolina at
    Chapel Hill
Chapel Hill, North Carolina

Connie N. Vance, Ed.D.
School of Nursing
College of New Rochelle
New Rochelle, New York

FORTHCOMING

ANNUAL REVIEW OF
NURSING RESEARCH, Volume 10

Tentative Contents

PART I
Research on Nursing Practice

Chapter 1

Arthritis

Vickie A. Lambert
MEDICAL COLLEGE OF GEORGIA

CONTENTS

Nurse researchers' interest in the examination of arthritis and its ramifications has been limited. Although nurses were interested in arthritis research and conducted studies throughout the 1970s and early 1980s, it was not until the mid-1980s that nurses' publications related to arthritis research began to increase. In this chapter, research conducted on arthritis by nurses is identified, described, and discussed and recommendations are presented for future research to enhance nursing's contributions to the field.

Arthritis refers to rheumatic diseases involving joint symptoms and abnormalities. By definition, arthritis means inflammation of the joint. However, the term often is used by the public to indicate any pain or stiffness of the musculoskeletal system whether or not the cause is an inflammatory process.

Of all chronic illnesses afflicting humans, none is more widespread and disabling than arthritis. Approximately 37 million people in the United States are afflicted with some type of arthritis. Of these individuals, approximately 8 million have rheumatoid arthritis, 18 million have osteoarthritis, 2.5 million have gout, and 8.5 million have various other types of arthritis and arthritis-

3

related afflictions (i.e., ankylosing spondylitis, psoratic arthritis, scleroderma, and systemic lupus arythematosis) (Metropolitan Washington Chapter of the Arthritis Foundation, 1986).

The Bureau of the Census estimates that approximately 18.9 million people have some form of limitation in activity as a result of arthritis (U.S. Department of Commerce, 1987). Because of its limiting effects, arthritis is a costly disease. Each year 26.6 billion work days are lost, $4.8 billion in wages are lost, $5 billion are spent on medical costs, and $1 billion are spent on disability aid and insurance (Metropolitan Washington Chapter of the Arthritis Foundation, 1986).

The cause of arthritis is unknown and, to date, there is no cure. However, it is possible to prevent, impede, or correct its crippling effects. Medications and surgical techniques often restore joint function and relieve pain. In addition, physical therapy is of value in relieving pain and preventing deformity.

To identify studies related to arthritis a search of the literature was conducted in several ways. A computerized search using MEDLINE for the years 1970 through 1988 was done using the subtitles of arthritis, nursing, and research. The *International Nursing Index* and the *Cumulative Index to Nursing and Allied Health Literature* were hand searched for the years 1970 through 1988, and the bibliographies of all retrieved articles were reviewed for the location of additional studies. The search was limited to sources published or in press in readily available journals and excluded abstracts and conference proceedings.

Studies included in the review were written in English and had a nurse as either the primary investigator or as one of the co-investigators. Studies that included a nurse who appeared to be a member of a medical research team were not included in the review. In addition, each study had as its focus a research question relevant to nursing science. Twenty-six studies were located.

Predominately two types of arthritis were examined in these studies: rheumatoid arthritis and osteoarthritis. The studies were categorized according to their research foci (a) psychosocial issues, (b) nursing intervention, (c) health care provider education, and (d) instrumentation issues.

NURSING RESEARCH RELATED TO ARTHRITIS PATIENTS

Psychosocial Issues

The majority of nurse investigators studying arthritis dealt with psychosocial issues related to the illness. Perhaps this was because psychosocial issues of illness commonly have been considered to be within nursing's domain. In this category, 17 studies were located that focused on six major aspects: well-being, quality of life, disease activity, causation, cost, and perceptions.

Well-being. The largest number of psychosocial studies ($N = 5$) were focused on a sense of well-being. Three of the studies were conducted by Lambert and associates (V. Lambert, 1985; V. Lambert & C. Lambert, 1985; V. Lambert, C. Lambert, Klipple, & Mewshaw, 1990). The general focus of the work of Lambert and colleagues was to analyze relationships of specific psychosocial variables to the dependent variable, psychological well-being, and to determine which combination of psychosocial variables was the best predictor of a sense of well-being in women with rheumatoid arthritis. In a study conducted in 1985, Lambert examined the relationship among social support, severity of illness, specific demographic characteristics, and psychological well-being. The findings suggested that pain, a measurement of illness severity, was the best predictor of psychological well-being. Because social support was not a predictor of well-being, V. Lambert and C. Lambert (1985) examined that relationship again in Caucasian and black women with rheumatoid arthritis. Low but significant correlations were found between each of the social support characteristics (affection, affirmation, and aid) and psychological well-being for Caucasian women, but not for black women. Using step-wise multiple regression analysis, as with V. Lambert's 1985 study, social support was not found to predict psychological well-being. V. Lambert and C. Lambert (1985) speculated that the nonsignificant findings were due to a lack of sufficient ethnic sensitivity of the evaluative instrument measuring social support. The low significant correlations found in Caucasian women and the lack of significant correlations found in black women may have been due to the small sample sizes ($n = 35$ and $n = 25$). A major limitation of the study was the lack of control for the level of illness severity among subjects. The level of rheumatoid arthritis severity possibily could have influenced a woman's ability to activate or use a social support system.

As a follow up of the two 1985 studies, V. Lambert and associates (1990) examined severity of illness, social support, and psychological hardiness as potential predictors of psychological well-being in women with rheumatoid arthritis. Using stepwise regression analysis, they found that satisfaction with social support and psychological hardiness, in that order, were significant predictors of well-being. Because one's level of illness severity may have influenced adaptation to the problems associated with rheumatoid arthritis, V. Lambert, C. Lambert, Klipple, and Mewshaw (1989) statistically controlled illness severity. Regardless of the level of illness severity, satisfaction with social support and psychological hardiness remained significant predictors of well-being in women with rheumatoid arthritis. The need to identify and empirically examine ways to foster both social support and hardiness with the intent of enhancing psychological well-being was supported by the findings.

To describe factors that promote adaptation, physiological, and psychosocial responses to chronic illness were measured by Pollock (1986). One of the chronic illnesses studied was rheumatoid arthritis. Pollock did not find a significant correlation between psychological hardiness and adaptation. Pollock's use of an investigator-constructed instrument to measure hardiness in addition to a small sample ($n = 20$) of individuals with rheumatoid arthritis may have contributed to the lack of significant findings.

As a means of examining well-being, Miller (1985) measured spiritual well-being and loneliness in healthy adults and in adults with rheumatoid arthritis. She hypothesized that: (a) there would be a negative correlation between loneliness and spiritual well-being in both healthy adults and adults with rheumatoid arthritis, (b) adults with rheumatoid arthritis would have significantly higher loneliness scores than healthy adults, and (c) adults with rheumatoid arthritis would have significantly lower spiritual well-being scores than healthy adults. The first hypothesis was supported, but not the second and third hypotheses. Miller speculated that the relationship between rheumatoid arthritis and loneliness was not supported because the instrument used to assess loneliness did not measure the multiple facets of the concept. Although the relationship between rheumatoid arthritis and spiritual well-being also was not supported, Miller suggested that this was the most significant finding of the study because high scores in spiritual well-being were found in both groups. In fact adults with rheumatoid arthritis had slightly higher spiritual well-being scores than healthy adults suggesting the importance of religious well-being to patients with a chronic illness. It must be kept in mind that this interpretation was not supported by the data but went beyond the findings. The findings of this study, however, must be viewed with caution because the groups differed considerably in age and gender composition. It is possible that age and gender could have influenced the study's findings.

Quality of Life.   In two studies, quality of life was examined. Laborde and Powers (1980, 1985) conducted two studies on individuals with osteoarthritis. The purpose of the 1980 study was to compare quality of life for patients undergoing hemodialysis to patients with severe osteoarthritis. The investigators found that patients undergoing hemodialysis perceived their present life as significantly more satisfying than did patients with osteoarthritis. In addition, dialysis patients viewed their present quality of life as better than their past life, whereas patients with osteoarthritis thought their present life quality was less satisfying than their past. Laborde and Powers suggested that their findings may have been the result of an increased sense of physical well-being experienced by the dialysis patients and the chronic pain experienced by patients with osteoarthritis.

As a follow up of their 1980 study, Laborde and Powers (1985) conducted a descriptive study to assess past, present, and future life satisfaction and to explore the relationships between perceived satisfaction with life, perceived health, health control orientation, and illness-related factors in individuals with osteoarthritis. The investigators reported that individuals rated their overall satisfaction with life and their recent health status as good. Present life satisfaction was related to perception of better health, internal health locus of control, and less arthritic joint pain. Laborde and Powers pointed out that such findings suggested the need for nurses planning health care goals for patients to keep in mind the osteoarthritic patient's orientation to the present. When generalizing Laborde and Powers findings, however, one must keep in mind that their sample was predominately Caucasian (79%), retired (67%), and female (77%).

Burkhardt (1985) explored the impact of pain and functional impairments on the quality of life experienced by individuals with arthritis. Using a cognitive framework, she developed a causal model in which disease-related variables interacting with demographic and social factors were hypothesized to affect quality of life indirectly through psychological mediators. The investigator reported that psychological mediators of positive self-esteem, internal control over health, perceived support, and low negative attitude toward the illness contributed directly to a higher quality of life. Severity of the arthritic impairment indirectly affected quality of life through the mediation of self-esteem and internal control over health. From Burkhardt's findings, self-esteem, a sense of personal control, and supportive relationships may have played major roles in influencing the perceptions of life satisfaction of individuals with arthritis. The fact that Burkhardt used subjects with various types of arthritis rather than one specific type could be perceived as a limitation in the study's design. The joints affected, the nature of the pain, and the physical mobility experienced by an individual often has depended on the type of arthritis present. Thus, psychological mediators that affected quality of life could have varied among individuals depending on the type of arthritis encountered.

To continue her examination of quality of life, Burkhardt (1988) compared the select aspects and satisfaction with those aspects between women in general and women with arthritis. Two hundred and twenty-five women with arthritis were compared to women from a randomly selected national population of women without arthritis. Burkhardt found that women with arthritis placed more importance on nonphysical recreational activity, on a close relationship with their spouse or significant other, and less importance on participating in governmental or local affairs. Women with arthritis were most satisfied with material comforts, relationships with relatives and close friends, helping and encouraging others, and nonphysical recreation than were women in general. Also, they were less satisfied with their health, work, and participation in physically active recreation than women in general. Burkhardt concluded that overall, women with arthritis were more similar to women within the general population than different from them. The significant differences in quality of life seemed to be attributed to arthritis. When generalizing Burkhardt's findings, however, one must consider the fact that the study subjects with arthritis were all middle class. This would have contributed to the subjects with arthritis ranking satisfaction with material comforts higher than subjects randomly selected from the general population of women.

Disease Activity.   Crosby (1988) studied the relationship among stress factors, emotional stress, and rheumatoid arthritic disease activity. She hypothesized that (a) there would be a positive correlation between emotional stress level and rheumatoid arthritis disease activity, and (b) there would be a positive correlation between the number and severity of stress factors and emotional stress level. Findings of the study supported both hypotheses. Crosby pointed out that the most important conclusion of her study was that emotional stress was related positively to rheumatoid arthritis disease activity. A major limitation in the study, however, was the use of an untested investigator-developed instrument for measuring rheumatoid arthritis disease activity. Thus the generalizability of the study's findings should be viewed with caution.

Causation.   Using a qualitative design, Elder (1974) identified explanations for the cause of osteoarthritic symptoms by men and women experiencing them and related those explanations to five social classes produced by socioeconomic status (i.e., occupation, education, and income). Higher social class subjects tended to state that aging, athletic injuries, stress, and heredity were most likely the causes of arthritic symptoms. Higher social class subjects also were more likely than lower social class subjects to refrain from giving any explanation for their symptoms, citing "don't know." Lower social class subjects gave climate, exposure to the elements, work conditions, work-related accidents, and punishment as likely causes of arthritic symptoms. Elder suggested that social class in the social structure influenced the explanations developed by individuals with arthritis to account for their symptoms. Since men and women in the lower classes were more likely to be engaged in physically active and traumatizing activities, they were more likely to offer these activities as arthritic symptoms. Elder's reporting of her findings would have been strengthened if she had more clearly delineated the details of her data collection process and data analysis and if she had more specifically related her findings to the five different social classes rather than simply describing class as higher and lower.

Lowery, Jacobsen, and Murphy (1983) linked causes of rheumatoid arthritis to behaviors, emotions, and expectations. Analysis of the data showed that although most subjects constructed causes to explain their arthritis, some did not. Individuals who had not constructed causes were significantly more anxious, more depressed, and more hostile than those who had. It was possible that persistence in using a noncausal way of thinking in situations of chronic illness, such as rheumatoid arthritis, eventually resulted in increased affective problems. In regard to attribution theory, Lowery and her colleagues showed that the causes given did not fit easily within the traditionally used classification model proposed by Weiner (1979). This, no doubt, was due to the fact that the model is based on the assumption that people *do* ascribe causes for life events. The uncertainty of chronic illness, however, may have evoked noncausal thinking as an adaptive response to the illness event.

Cost. As part of a one year longitudinal study, Spitz (1984) examined the medical, personal, and social costs of rheumatoid arthritis to patients living in Northern California. Costs to the patients were calculated in dollar expenditures, lost work days, indication of the most significant consequence of the arthritic disease process, and changes in lifestyle. Spitz reported that the largest outpatient costs were for medications and physicians' fees, that pain was the most significant consequence of the disease, and that autonomy in the workplace and income prior to disease onset were the most significant factors influencing lost work days. A multitude of ways that rheumatoid arthritis can affect a patient and his or her family were identified in Spitz's findings.

Perceptions. In a descriptive study by Wright and Hopkins (1977), rheumatic patients, nurses, and physicians were asked to interpret the meaning of 30 words related to anatomy, symptoms, diseases, and treatment. Findings showed that only two terms, heredity and rheumatism, held the same meaning for patients, nurses, and physicians. Major differences in word meanings existed between patients and physicians for (a) symptoms—numbness; (b) parts of the body—spinal cord, cervical, sacrum, and loin; (c) disorders—slipped disc, arthritis, osteoarthritis, and (d) treatment—steroids. In regard to patients and nurses, major differences in word meanings existed for anemia, cervical, and sacrum. There was agreement on the meaning of words between physicians and nurses. Wright and Hopkins pointed out the importance of using terms carefully when explaining situations to patients.

Lorig, Cox, Cuevas, Kraines, and Britton (1984) conducted a survey of Caucasian patients, Spanish-speaking patients, and physicians regarding salient beliefs about arthritis and treatment. Findings were: (a) beliefs of Caucasian patients and physicians were similar, (b) physicians generally underestimated the knowledge and beliefs of their patients about traditional proven treatments, and (c) physicians overestimated patients' beliefs in nontraditional therapies. Caucasian and Spanish-speaking patients held divergent beliefs about treatments for arthritis and about factors that would worsen arthritis symptoms. The comparsion of the Caucasian patients and the

Spanish-speaking patients should be viewed with caution, however, because there was a major educational difference between the two groups and the study design did not provide for confirmation of arthritis in the Spanish-speaking patients as in the Caucasian patients. The findings illustrated the importance of physicians and other health care providers addressing patients' beliefs about arthritis.

Two sets of nurse researchers (Muhlenkamp & Joyner, 1986; Taylor, Passo, & Champion, 1987) compared perceptions of patients with arthritis and perceptions of others regarding issues surrounding arthritis. Muhlenkamp and Joyner (1986) examined differences between arthritis patients' self-reported affective states (anxiety, hostility, and depression) and nurses' perceptions of patients' affective states. The investigators found that nurse caregivers generally were accurate in their assessment of arthritic patients' affective states. Of additional interest were the findings that nurse caregivers' attribution of anxiety was correlated positively with the patient's socioeconomic status and that the higher the educational level of the nurse, the more accurate was his or her assessment. The only demographic variable positively correlated to the patient's self report of anxiety and depression was the number of patient hospitalizations encountered.

Taylor and associates (1987) compared perceptions of children who had juvenile rheumatoid arthritis with perceptions of their parents and teachers regarding the frequency of potential school problems and their opinions regarding the extent of the teacher's responsibility in helping children to deal with medical, academic, or social issues. Findings showed that children felt that problems with self-concept and peer relationships occurred more frequently, whereas parents and teachers believed that physical health and activity-related problems were more prevalent. Childrens' ratings regarding the extent of a teacher's responsibility in helping them were lower than those of parents' or teachers' ratings. Although parents and teachers viewed teachers as being responsible for helping children deal with psychosocial-related issues, children believed that teachers should deal primarily with academic issues. Based on their findings, Taylor and associates emphasized the importance of considering children's views about school problems and teachers' responsibilities in dealing with these problems before initiating interventions.

Nursing Interventions

The second largest number of nursing studies conducted on arthritis dealt with nursing interventions. Five of the intervention studies were related to patient education and one to exercise.

In a study of 200 individuals with arthritis, Lorig, Lauren, and Holman (1984) examined the longitudinal effects of a 12-hour community-based, lay-led arthritis self-management course on knowledge, pain, disability, and number of visits to the physician. Subjects in the 55 to 74 age group showed, after the course, significant gain in knowledge, diminished pain for 20 months, and decreases in disability for 8 months. Subjects in the 75 to 94 age group also increased their knowledge for 20 months and decreased their pain and the number of visits to physicians for 8 months after the course. Two limitations of the study's design were the arbitrary decision to divide the subjects into two age groups with 74 years being the cut off point and the small sample size of the 75 to 94 age group ($n = 43$) in comparison to the 55 to 74 age group ($n = 152$).

To build on the knowledge gained from the 1984 study, Lorig, Lubeck, Kraines, Seleznick, and Holman (1985) conducted a longitudinal experimental study to address the outcomes of a lay-led arthritis self-management course. In a randomized experiment testing a 4-month intervention, experimental subjects at 4 months exceeded control subjects in knowledge, lessened pain, and the practice of self-management behaviors. These significant findings remained at 20 months. A strength of the study design was the use of an experimental design with measurement of the dependent variables over an extended period of time. The findings of the two studies conducted by Lorig et al. (1984) and Lorig, Lubeck, et al. (1985) reflect the influence of a formal course of instruction on the growth of knowledge and adoption of taught behaviors over an extended period of time.

The effects of self-instruction on learning, satisfaction with self-instruction, and health status of persons with rheumatoid arthritis were examined by Oermann, Doyle, Clark, River, and Rose (1986). They hypothesized that compared to patients who received no structured teaching, patients who completed a self-instructional program would: (a) learn significantly more, (b) demonstrate satisfaction with the teaching method, and (c) demonstrate greater improvement in their perceived health status. The findings supported the first and second hypotheses, but not the third. Oermann and colleagues believed that knowledge of one's illness and the ability to perform self-care measures may not have been sufficient in influencing health status if the client's rheumatoid arthritis condition failed to improve or if the client refused to comply with his or her treatment regimen.

Laborde and Powers (1983) conducted an experimental study in which they evaluated five educational interventions focused on pain and disease management in a variety of settings for individuals with osteoarthritis. The interventions included provision of: (a) an information brochure; (b) joint preservation teaching plus a brochure; (c) relaxation procedure plus the brochure; (d) relaxation procedure, joint preservation teaching, and the brochure; and (e) no treatment. Effectiveness of each intervention was determined by measures of pain, stiffness, amount of medication, mobility, change in perceived level of pain-related stress, and knowledge gained about osteoarthritis. No single education intervention for osteoarthritis management showed sufficient patient benefit to support adoption into routine nursing practice. It is possible that significant findings were not shown because only 35 subjects were in each of the first four educational intervention groups and 20 were in the control group.

Conine, Carty, and Wood-Johnson (1987) conducted a survey using matched pairs of primiparous women with rheumatoid arthritis and physically functional nonrheumatoid arthritis controls to identify and compare the nature and source of childbirth education received by the two groups and the deficiencies in the education as perceived by the subjects. They found that less than 50% of each group received adequate professional information on childbirth and that significantly more of the women with rheumatoid arthritis reported their childbirth education needs were not met satisfactorily. In addition, the primaparous women with rheumatoid arthritis received information primarily from a lay person instead of a professional health care provider. The findings of the study, however, must be viewed with caution because no information was collected regarding the type of health care delivery system used by either the rheumatoid arthritis patients or the physically functional nonrheumatoid arthritis controls. The type of health care delivery system used by a subject could have influenced decidedly the type and quality of the childbirth education received.

Only one study was located in which researchers tested interventions not related to patient education. The purpose of the quasi-experimental study conducted by Byers (1985) was to test the effects of evening exercises on morning stiffness and joint mobility of the right index finger in patients with rheumatoid arthritis. As hypothesized, the performance of evening exercises resulted in less stiffness than when evening exercises were not performed. Patients in the lower end of the stiffness range, however, did not perceive subjectively an effect of evening exercises as great as did patients in the upper end of the range. As anticipated, finger mobility was greater when evening exercises were performed and after morning exercises. The findings of this study would have relevance for planning exercises involving the right index finger; however, replication and extension of the design would be required for generalization to exercises involving joints in other parts of the body.

Health Care Provider Education

Two experimental studies (Mazzuca, Barger, & Brandt, 1987; Small & Martinson, 1987) were located in which investigators addressed educational programs for health care providers related to arthritis. The underlying premise of the studies was that an educational program should influence providers' behavior with respect to the delivery of health care.

Mazzuca and colleagues (1987) evaluated an inservice training program for public health nurses (PHN) who were on staff at one of seven older-adult clinics. The purpose of the study was to compare control group peers with public health nurses who received an inservice education program about arthritis in older adults. It was hypothesized that nurses in the inservice education group would screen their clients more frequently for joint pain, joint swelling, and limitations in ambulation and activities of daily living, and would follow the program's recommendation more frequently for the management of identified arthritis-related problems. The researchers reported that the inservice education program was successful in producing significant differences between the groups with respect to screening for common arthritis-related problems, but not successful in fostering the implementation of management practices related to arthritis problems. Mazzuca et al. suggested that the unsuccessful implementation of management practices following the inservice program was due to the nurses' primary concern during the early phases of the inservice educational program about administering seasonal influenza inoculations to patients rather than concern about changing their habitual practice patterns. Usefulness of the study's findings was limited because the inservice education group ($n = 21$) was approximately twice the size of the comparison group ($n = 8$), the criteria for subject inclusion were not described, and the assessment of the subject's responses to the inservice educational program was made by an unqualified individual.

In a randomized experimental study, Small and Martinson (1987) investigated the effectiveness of an inservice education program for home health aides on the transmittal of information to patients about ways to manage activities of daily living more effectively. No significant differences were found between groups. Small and Martinson speculated that the findings were influenced by the lack of professional supervision of the aides and the lack of patient receptivity to the transmittal of information by nonprofessional personnel. It also was likely that the study showed insignificant findings because the size of both the experimental ($n = 5$) and the control groups ($n = 9$) was very small. The insignificant findings in both studies regarding the effect of an educational program on the health care providers' delivery of care most likely were due to the flaws in both studies' designs.

Instrumentation Issues

The only located study to address issues of instrumentation was conducted by Goeppinger, Doyle, Charlton, and Lorig (1988), whose purpose was to examine the psychometric properties of two self-administered measures of function: the disability score of the Health Assessment Questionnaire (HAQ) (Fries, Spitz, & Young, 1982) and the total health score of the Arthritis Impact Measurement Scales (AIMS) (Meenan, Gertman, & Mason, 1980). Reliabilities (test–retest and internal consistency) and concurrent validity ranged from moderate to high in both measures. Content analysis suggested that the HAQ may be more appropriate than the AIMS for use with rural residents and that it may reflect, more comprehensively, areas of function relevant to nursing practice.

RESEARCH CONTRIBUTIONS

The majority of studies addressing arthritis were focused on psychosocial factors and nursing interventions. Few researchers have dealt with physiological aspects, health care provider education, and instrumentation.

Investigators who studied psychosocial issues predominately have contributed knowledge to understanding of (a) types of factors that influence ability to cope with the problems related to arthritis, (b) factors that enhance one's ability to foster quality of life, and (c) individuals' perceptions about arthritis. Few investigators have examined psychosocial factors and disease activity, beliefs of disease causation, psychological and social costs of disease, and health care issues related to children.

The majority of studies conducted on psychosocial factors have been descriptive, they included a survey design, and valid and reliable instruments to measure the variables. Limitations evident across several studies were (a) small sample sizes, (b) lack of multiple measures to assess severity of the arthritic disease process, (c) lack of control for level of illness severity among subjects, (d) the use of subjects in a single study who have various types of arthritis, and (e) the use of noncomparable groups.

Researchers testing nursing interventions have contributed additional information on the usefulness of several educational approaches and on the use of exercise to enhance mobility. An insufficient number of studies have been conducted to support the adoption of any one type of educational or exercise approach for use with individuals with arthritis. The intervention studies have incorporated experimental or quasi-experimental designs. The limitations across studies in this category included: (a) small sample sizes, (b) limited generalizability, (c) arbitrary decision making in the creation of subject groups, and (d) lack of control of intervening variables.

In the two studies conducted on health care provider education, investigators examined educational programs in regard to changing providers' behavior with respect to delivery of health care. Findings from one study

Mazzuca et al., 1987) indicated that an inservice education program produced change in providers' screening activities for common arthritis related problems. Most of the research findings in this category were insignificant, most likely because of flaws in the designs of the studies, including (a) unequal sized groups, (b) unqualified subject evaluators, and (c) small sample sizes.

The one located study of instrumentation contributed knowledge about two measures of function, the disability score of the Health Assessment Questionnaire (Fries et al., 1982) and the total health score of the Arthritis Impact Measurement Scale (Meenan et al., 1980). The fact that only one study could be found that addressed instrumentation issues indicated the great void of nursing research in this area. Because assessment of physiological function has been a necessity for determining severity of illness in individuals with arthritis, continued research in this area would be important. In addition, the development of new instruments that measure psychosocial parameters related to arthritis should occur.

RECOMMENDATIONS FOR FUTURE RESEARCH

A number of recommendations are made to enhance the contributions of nursing research in the field of arthritis care. First, there should be an increase in the number of longitudinal studies conducted. Arthritis is a chronic disease that evolves over time, and most nurse researchers have examined only one point in time in the life of an individual with arthritis. Studies are needed that incorporate repeated measures over time of both physiologic and psychosocial variables in order to enable better understanding of the types of changes that occur and to identify the patterns that exist in those changes.

More studies are needed to test a variety of educational methods for use with patients, significant others, and health care providers in regard to arthritis care. Because no one method of education has been identified as being the most effective, ongoing assessment of educational approaches with subjects of different ages and with different types of arthritis should occur.

No studies were located that addressed health promotion or illness prevention related to arthritis. This is a fertile field for nursing research.

Researchers have only begun to identify and study variables empirically that predict psychological well-being and quality of life in persons with arthritis. Additional studies in this field should address a wider range of both physiologic and psychosocial variables. These studies should include a focus on the severity of illness experienced by subjects to understand how severity influences other aspects of health and treatment. When the severity of the arthritic disease process is measured, it should include the assessment of multiple parameters, in addition to pain. Although pain is one of the most accurate indicators of disease activity, it is not the *only* one. Such measurements as joint function, length of morning stiffness, and physical mobility are but a few additional indicators that can be assessed.

Studies are needed to address problems related to children and their parents. A child's level of development should be taken into consideration in the design of future studies because coping processes used by a child and nursing interventions will vary depending on the child's state of development.

Empirical studies of specific nursing interventions related to both physiologic and psychosocial care are needed. Only one study testing a nursing intervention other than educational instruction was located. To prescribe adequate nursing care for patients with arthritis, nursing interventions must be founded on sound research.

The identification of perceived needs of patients and their significant others is lacking. Research questions focusing on this area should be addressed so that nursing is assessing correctly the health care needs of the individual with arthritis and his or her family.

Studies that examine physiologic responses are needed such as the identification of personal and environmental factors that might contribute to or prevent the remission and exacerbation of the arthritic process. No studies could be located on this topic.

Finally, to have research findings that are reliable and valid, sound instruments to measure appropriate variables are needed. Studies to develop new instruments and examine their psychometric properties are essential, as are studies to determine the psychometric properties of existing instruments. The field of research in arthritis care is fertile for nurses. Many avenues for research questions remain open and unexplored. The time is right for nursing to make its mark!

REFERENCES

Burkhardt, C. (1985). The impact of arthritis on quality of life. *Nursing Research, 34,* 11–16.

Burkhardt, C. (1988). Quality of life for women with arthritis. *Health Care for Women International, 9,* 229–238.

Byers, P. (1985). Effect of exercise on morning stiffness and mobility in patients with rheumatoid arthritis. *Research in Nursing & Health, 8,* 275–281.

Conine, T., Carty, E., & Wood-Johnson, F. (1987). Nature and source of information received by primiparas with rheumatoid arthritis on preventive maternal and child care. *Canadian Journal of Public Health, 78,* 393–397.

Crosby, L. (1988). Stress factors, emotional stress, and rheumatoid arthritis disease activity. *Journal of Advanced Nursing, 13,* 452–461.

Elder, R. (1974). Social class and lay explanations of the etiology of arthritis. *Nursing Digest, 2,* 23–31.

Fries, J., Spitz, P., & Young, D. (1982). The dimensions of health outcomes: The Health Assessment Questionnaire, disability and pain scales. *The Journal of Rheumatology, 9,* 789–793.

Goeppinger, J., Doyle, A., Charlton, S., & Lorig, K. (1988). A nursing perspective on the assessment of function in persons with arthritis. *Research in Nursing and Health, 11,* 321–331.

Laborde, J., & Powers, M. (1980). Satisfaction with life for patients undergoing hemodialysis and patients suffering from osteoarthritis. *Research in Nursing & Health, 3,* 19–24.

Laborde, J., & Powers, M. (1983). Evaluation of educational interventions for osteoarthritics. *Multiple Linear Regression Viewpoints, 12,* 12–37.

Laborde, J., & Powers, M. (1985). Life satisfaction, health control, orientation, and illness-related factors in persons with osteoarthritis. *Research in Nursing & Health, 8,* 183–190.

Lambert, V. (1985). Study of factors associated with psychological well-being in rheumatoid arthritic women. *Image: The Journal of Nursing Scholarship, 17,* 50–53.

Lambert, V., & Lambert, C. (1985). The relationship between social support and psychological well-being in rheumatoid arthritic women from two ethnic groups. *Health Care for Women International, 6,* 405–414.

Lambert, V., Lambert, C., Klipple, G., & Mewshaw, E. (1990). A study of the relationships among hardiness, social support, severity of illness, and psychological well-being in women with rheumatoid arthritis. *Health Care for Women International, 11,* 159–173.

Lambert, V., Lambert, C., Klipple, G., & Mewshaw, E. (1989). Psychosocial factors predicting psychological well-being in women with rheumatoid arthritis when severity of illness is statistically controlled. *Image: The Journal of Nursing Scholarship, 21,* 128–133.

Lorig, K., Cox, T., Cuevas, X., Kraines, R., & Britton, M. (1984). Converging and diverging beliefs about arthritis: Caucasian patients, Spanish speaking patients, and physicians. *Journal of Rheumatology, 11,* 76–79.

Lorig, K., Lauren, J., & Holman, H. (1984). Arthritis self-management: A study of the effectiveness of patient education for the elderly. *Gerontologist, 24,* 455–457.

Lorig, K., Lubeck, D., Kraines, R., Seleznick, M., & Holman, H. (1985). Outcomes of self-help and education for patients with arthritis. *Arthritis and Rheumatism, 28,* 680–685.

Lowery, B., Jacobsen, B., & Murphy, B. (1983). An exploratory investigation of causal thinking of arthritics. *Nursing Research, 32,* 157–162.

Mazzuca, S., Barger, G., & Brandt, K. (1987). Arthritis care in older-adult centers: A controlled study of an education program for public health nurses. *Arthritis and Rheumatism, 30,* 275–280.

Meenan, R., Gertman, P., & Mason, J. (1980). Measuring health status in arthritis: The Arthritis Impact Measurement Scales. *Arthritis and Rheumatism, 23,* 146–151.

Metropolitan Washington Chapter of the Arthritis Foundation. (1986). *Fact sheet on arthritis.* Arlington, VA: Author.

Miller, J. (1985). Assessment of loneliness and spiritual well-being in chronically ill and healthy adults. *Journal of Professional Nursing, 1,* 79–85.

Muhlenkamp, A., & Joyner, J. (1986). Arthritis patients' self-reported affective states and their caregivers' perceptions. *Nursing Research, 35,* 24–27.

Oermann, M., Doyle, T., Clark, L., River, C., & Rose, V. (1986). Effectiveness of self-instruction for arthritis patient education. *Patient Education and Counseling, 8,* 245–254.

Pollock, S. (1986). Human responses to chronic illness: Physiologic and psychosocial adaptation. *Nursing Research, 35,* 90–95.

Small, D., & Martinson, I. (1987). In-service training of home health aides for arthritis care. *Journal of Community Health Nursing, 4,* 243–251.

Spitz, P. (1984). The medical, personal, and social costs of rheumatoid arthritis. *Nursing Clinics of North America, 19,* 575–582.

Taylor, J., Passo, M., & Champion, V. (1987). School problems and teacher responsibilities in juvenile rheumatoid arthritis. *Journal of School Health, 57,* 186–190.

U.S. Department of Commerce, Bureau of the Census. (1987). *Statistical abstract of the United States.* Washington, DC: Author.

Weiner, B. (1979). Theory of motivation for some classroom experiences. *Journal of Education Psychology, 71,* 3–25.

Wright, V. & Hopkins, R. (1977). Communicating with the rheumatic patient. *Nursing Times, 73,* 1308–1313.

Chapter 2

Alzheimer's Disease

MERIDEAN L. MAAS
COLLEGE OF NURSING
THE UNIVERSITY OF IOWA

KATHLEEN C. BUCKWALTER
COLLEGE OF NURSING
THE UNIVERSITY OF IOWA

CONTENTS

In 1907 Alois Alzheimer delineated a syndrome that remained in virtual obscurity until the past decade. Long attributed to senility, hardening of the arteries, or the aging process, Senile Dementia of the Alzheimer's Type or Alzheimer's disease (AD) is now a household word. Approximately 10% of persons between the ages of 65 and 75 years and 25% of those over 85 are reported to suffer some form of dementia (Evans et al., 1989). Sixty percent of the elderly who are demented are reported to have Alzheimer's disease

(Fryer, 1983; Pajik, 1984). Also, as the percentage of older Americans increases from 11.3% in 1980 to 21.6% by the year 2040, the number of cases of Alzheimer's disease is expected to quintuple (Office of Technology Assessment [OTA], 1987). The costs of Alzheimer's disease are enormous. Direct costs to society are estimated to be $38 billion per year, and total costs, which include indirect expenditures, exceed $88 billion per year (Blass, 1990).

It is mostly within the past 10 years that nurse scientists have conducted investigations in this area. Although the number of nursing studies continues to be small compared to medical research efforts, reported nursing studies in Alzheimer's disease are increasing rapidly. Overall, the total number of indexed publications on dementia has grown from 87 in 1976 to 548 in 1985, corresponding to the increase in resources allocated to Alzheimer's disease research from less than 4 million dollars in 1976 to more than 50 million dollars in 1986 (OTA, 1987). The majority of this research has been biomedical, with studies focused on discovery of the pathological etiology of Alzheimer's disease and on pharmaceutical interventions to eliminate or ease the signs and symptoms. Nursing research questions have received much less attention than biomedical and basic research efforts, despite the need to develop knowledge concerning the antecedents and consequences of nursing diagnoses associated with Alzheimer's disease and the approaches that promote quality of life for Alzheimer's disease victims and their families. As knowledge of the disease, diagnosis, prognosis, and interventions has developed through research, the nurse's role in the management of Alzheimer's disease has evolved, although supporting research has not been available consistently. Nurses now assume major responsibilities for assessment, diagnosis, and management of nursing problems along the entire care continuum in Alzheimer's disease patients. Once the diagnosis of Alzheimer's disease has been made, the care required by the Alzheimer's disease patient and family is primarily nursing.

Overall, nursing studies in Alzheimer's disease are scattered over a range of topics, often with one or two research reports addressing the same questions. Because of this an integrated review of nursing research in Alzheimer's disease is difficult. Wherever possible, we have attempted to identify research findings, strengths, and weaknesses of the several isolated studies.

A review of the literature was conducted in all healthcare journals using Selected Dissemination of Information (SDI), MEDLINE, and quarterly AGELINE searches covering the past decade (from 1979 through early 1990). Additional articles were located from the references listed in research articles and through correspondence with nurses who are known experts in gerontology and mental health.

A nurse had to be first author or a contributing author and member of a research team for an article to be included in the review. Many articles that appeared to meet this criterion, upon review, were not research or data-based. It was often difficult to determine from citations and manuscripts if authors published in nonnursing journals were nurses; thus, some key nursing studies in Alzheimer's disease that were being published during the time the chapter was written may have been missed. Over 70 articles by nurses reporting empirical data were found. Following a brief overview of the disease, the chapter is organized by the nature of the problems of care and nursing interventions within subheadings of the continuum of care and settings.

DEMENTIA OF THE ALZHEIMER'S TYPE

There are many classifications of the over 70 different conditions that cause dementia of middle and later ages (Blass, 1982; Katzman, 1986). A distinction should be made between dementias of reversible or irreversible etiologies. If a reversible dementia is determined, medical treatment often can restore normal function. If an irreversible dementia is diagnosed, it is important to distinguish further among a number of etiologies that result in cognitive and behavioral changes that are quite similar. The inability to definitively diagnose Alzheimer's disease, except at autopsy, makes differential diagnosis difficult.

Alzheimer's disease is the most common of the irreversible, degenerative dementias, accounting for about 60% of the 3 to 4 million Americans diagnosed with dementing illness (Cross & Gurland, 1986). Alzheimer's disease is a progressive degenerative disorder of unknown etiology. The diagnosis of Alzheimer's disease is made by exclusion of other possible causes of dementia (McKhann et al., 1984). The concept of person-environment fit described in nursing is derived from systems theory and emphasizes the inter-relatedness of systems and their subsystems (Lawton, 1975a) and has been used by nurses and others to explain AD patient behavior and to propose management strategies. Dysfunctional and socially inappropriate behavior of Alzheimer's disease patients can be more easily understood in terms of person–environment fit, in that impairment of ego-sensory, perceptual, and cognitive processes affect overall ability to interact successfully with the environment (Silverstone & Burach-Weiss, 1983).

The person–environment interaction model has roots in the person–environment fit perspective and is also prominent in understanding and guiding the function and care of persons with Alzheimer's disease, focusing on the interaction of cognitive function and environmental characteristics (Hogstel, 1979; Kahana, 1975; Lawton, 1975b). Due to cognitive impairment, the Alzheimer's disease patient exhibits behaviors that indicate disordered person–environment interaction: repetitive behaviors, catastrophic reactions, and situationally inappropriate behaviors (Roberts & Algase, 1988).

Much care has been based on the notion that Alzheimer's disease patients need increased environmental stimuli to correct cognitive and functional deficits (Doyle, Dunn, Thadani, & Lenihan, 1986; Gillies, 1986; Ridder, 1985; Wolanin & Phillips, 1981); however, most interventions from this perspective have not been successful (Lawton, 1980; Peterson, Knapp, Rosen, & Pither, 1977; Woods, 1982). Rather, there is some evidence that Alzheimer's disease patients spontaneously attempt to reduce environmental stimuli by isolating themselves from other persons (DeLong, 1970; Maxwell, Bader, & Watson, 1972).

Hall and Buckwalter (1987) proposed that Alzheimer's disease patients need environmental demands modified because of their declining abilities and described the Progressively Lowered Threshold Model to guide nursing interventions and as an heuristic model for research. In the model, the increasing inability of the person with Alzheimer's disease to cope with stress due to the progressive cerebral pathology and associated cognitive decline is described (Hall & Buckwalter, 1987). Stress from environmental and internal demands causes the Alzheimer's disease patient to be anxious. If the stressful stimuli are allowed to continue or increase, the patient's behavior becomes increasingly dysfunctional and often catastrophic, that is, suddenly occurring emotional behavioral responses that are out of proportion to the stimulus, indicating cognitive and social inaccessability. Thus the Progressively Lowered Threshold model reduces stress by modifying environmental demands, thereby promoting functional adaptive behavior on the part of the Alzheimer's disease client.

Disordered person–environment interactions also result when the family caregiver can no longer cope with care in the home. Family caregiving tends to continue following institutionalization of the relative (Wilson, 1989). Thus, the progressively deteriorating clinical course of Alzheimer's disease necessitates role transition and adjustment for family members along several dimensions: (a) primary caregiver to visitor, (b) insider to outsider, and (c) high control to low control over the patient's care priorities. When the Alzheimer's disease patient is institutionalized, staff caregivers assume the primary caregiving role and are the insiders with high control over the priorities of care. Therefore, the relationship between family members and institutional caregivers may be problematic, limiting the quality of patient care (Pratt, Schmall, Wright, & Hare, 1987). Difficulties with adjustment for family members and Alzheimer's disease patients may be due to (a) conflict with staff over the caregiver role and the frequency and length of family member visits, (b) disagreements over the use of formal services, (c) family member criticism of the care provided by staff, and (d) the person with Alzheimer's disease becoming upset during visits by family members.

The person-environment interaction perspective identifies institutional barriers (e.g., structures, policies, regulations, attitudes, and behaviors) that are not responsive to family members' needs as well as those resources that help family members maintain involvement in the patient's care (Buckwalter & Hall, 1987). The model addresses these issues in an effort to reduce institutional barriers that can often interfere with satisfying family member participation in the Alzheimer's disease patient's care (Buckwalter & Hall, 1987).

Through these theoretical frameworks nurses have emphasized the relationship of the person and the environment. The frameworks support environmental and behavioral management as a major focus of nursing interventions. Although these theoretical frameworks are promising, more research is needed to test the models that shape understanding of the care of persons with Alzheimer's disease and their families and guide nursing practice and research efforts.

NURSING ASSESSMENT

Cognitive Status

Although there are nursing assessment tools designed to help the nurse more accurately describe cognitive status, only a few have been systematically evaluated for reliability and validity. Palmateer and McCartney (1985) compared nursing assessment techniques with the use of the Cognitive Capacity Screening Examination to measure the cognitive status of hospitalized medical-surgical patients over age 65. Nursing assessments did not include formal cognitive testing or enough precise behavioral descriptions and failed to identify a significant number of cognitively impaired elderly when compared to those identified by the Cognitive Capacity Screen Examination.

Confusion

Wolanin and Phillips (1981) delineated five categories of sources of confusion: (1) compromised brain support, (2) sensoriperceptual problems, (3) disruption in pattern and meaning, (4) alterations in normal physiologic states, and (5) the true dementias. These categories were used as the conceptual framework for a study of nursing home personnel's knowledge and opinions about reversible and irreversible forms of confusion (Lincoln, 1984). All nursing staff had a high percentage of incorrect responses about irreversible dementia, particularly Alzheimer's disease, although there was a positive linear relationship between knowledge of the sources of confusion and the amount of formal education for both licensed and nonlicensed nursing staff.

To describe confusion based on caregivers' perceptions, a study was conducted that included 30 elderly persons (age > 65) whom the staff labeled as confused (Wolanin & Phillips, 1981). Data were gathered from nurses' and physicians' records and taped interviews with staff. Physicians tended to view confusion as a symptom related to a pathological state that is reversible, whereas nurses labeled elderly as confused when they had both irreversible and reversible brain pathology.

Much of the nursing literature on acute confusional states is devoted to management of delirium (Batt, 1989; Campbell, Williams & Mlynarczyk, 1986), or differentiation of delirium from dementia (Gomez & Gomez, 1989). Nursing research related to delirium has been focused on patients in acute care, rather than long-term care settings (Chisholm, Deniston, Igrisam, & Barbus, 1982; Foreman, 1986).

Sundown Syndrome

Sundown syndrome is defined as confusion that either occurs or increases in the late afternoon or evening hours around sunset (Evans, 1987). To describe sundown syndrome, its prevalence in a population of nursing home residents, and related psychosocial, physiologic, and environmental factors, Evans (1987) studied 59 demented and 30 nondemented institutionalized older persons. The majority of patients were black, single, and their mean age was 80 years. A battery of standardized and investigator-developed psychosocial and mental status instruments were used along with physiologic, psychosocial, environmental, and sensory screening data. Reliability and validity of these instruments were reported by Evans. Increased restlessness and verbal behavior around sunset was associated with greater cognitive impairment, dehydration, being awakened more frequently at night for nursing care, more recent admission to the facility, and residing in their present room less than one month. However, 85% of the demented patients showed no symptoms of sundown syndrome. There was no statistically significant relationship with morale, medications, demographic variables or increased use of physical restraints in the evening, and sundowners had fewer diagnosed medical disorders than nonsundowners. Evans (1987) identified the need for more comprehensive research with around-the-clock observations of sleep-wake behavior and with more exact indicators of depression, hydration, and biological rhythms.

Functional Status

Although the average length of time from diagnosis of Alzheimer's disease to death is 7 to 10 years (Jolles & Hijman, 1983), Alzheimer's disease patients vary greatly in their lifespan and in the progressive loss of functional abilities. The need for descriptive research to identify early and late changes in functioning of persons with Alzheimer's disease has been noted (Cohen, Kennedy, & Eisdorfer, 1984). Although there has been little nursing research in this area, Booth, Bradley, and Whall (1988) used historical data from family reports at the time of diagnosis to describe premorbid, early, and late changes in functioning of persons with Alzheimer's disease. Survey findings from 46 surrogate respondents suggested a marked decline in intellectual, social, and self-care functioning from the premorbid to the early stage of Alzheimer's disease. Problems with work, organization of life activities, grooming, and self-care predominated. From early to advanced stages of the disease, verbal and nonverbal communication abilities, performance of tasks, and bowel and bladder control declined most. In the later stages, about 80% of the subjects had choreoform movements and about half were nonambulatory. Selected functional declines in the premorbid stage need further attention and have important implications for preventive nursing interventions.

The development and testing of comprehensive functional assessment instruments in which researchers incorporate perceptual, cognitive, and environmental components has received little attention in the nursing research literature. Noting that instruments to measure activites of daily living were developed to assess physical function and were not designed to assess cognitive dysfunctions that influence self-care abilities, Beck (1988) designed and tested a Dressing Performance Scale for use with persons with dementia. Following a task analysis of dressing behavior based on multiple observations of demented persons and caregivers, a hierarchy of types of caregiver assistance was defined. These categories of assistance included: (a) no assistance, (b) stimulus control, (c) initial verbal prompt, (d) gestures or modeling, (e) occasional physical guidance, (f) complete physical guidance, and (g) complete assistance.

Sandman, Norberg, Adolfsson, Axelsson, and Hedly (1986) studied 5 hospitalized patients with Alzheimer's disease to describe the behaviors of patients and nurses during morning care. All subjects were severly demented and required some assistance. A 12-step classification scheme was developed to use as a guide to understand and determine abilities essential for performance of morning care for demented patients. The results shed light on the complexity of providing nursing assistance for this stressful self-care task. The research found that missing abilities could be determined, that highest level of performance varied from day to day, and that the nurse could compensate for the Alzheimer's disease patient's fragmented behavior. Apraxia was identified as the critical factor in morning care. Paratonia (increasing muscle tone during passive movements of different strength) was frequently observed, a response that could be falsely interpreted as conscious resistance or refusal to participate.

In an experimental study to evaluate the effects of a Special Alzheimer's Unit (SU) on Alzheimer's disease patients' functional status, Maas and Buckwalter (1990) developed and tested a Functional Abilities Checklist (FAC). The instrument was developed because existing measures did not address all of the behaviors of demented patients that influence their abilities to function in their environment. The 5 areas included in the FAC are: self-care abilities; inappropriate behaviors; cognitive status; agitation behaviors; and sexual behaviors. This instrument has undergone extensive psychometric evaluation with data from the Maas and Buckwalter research program. Doyle et al. (1986) pilot tested the CADET (which measures communication, ambulation, daily activity, elimination, and transfer) (Rameizl, 1983) and FROMAJE (which measures function, reason, orientation, memory, arithmetic, judgement, and emotions) (Libow, 1981) instruments to assess Alzheimer's disease patients on a special care Alzheimer's unit and found them useful in determining mental and physical functional abilities, although further evaluation of reliability and validity was recommended.

EVALUATION OF NURSING ASSESSMENT RESEARCH

Cognitive changes resulting in memory loss and confusion are classic symptoms of Alzheimer's disease. However, confusion can be acute or chronic. To meet the special needs of Alzheimer's disease patients, nurses must be able to assess cognitive capacity and to distinguish reversible from irreversible etiologies. As the management of associated behaviors for reversible and irreversible dementias can be very different, there is a need to conduct research on the phenomenon of delirium and confusion in both acute and long-term care settings, and to investigate assessment and management strategies when the two conditions co-exist in persons in a variety of settings.

The effects of nursing interventions on sundown syndrome should be studied. Research is also needed to determine whether sundown syndrome is a unique phenomenon, distinguishable from other types of confusion or if it is associated with specific behaviors and characteristics of irreversibly demented patients.

Nursing research is needed to develop and test comprehensive functional assessment tools and tools to measure specific deficits so that targeted nursing interventions can be designed to assist demented persons to remain as functionally able as possible. Adaptation of existing functional assessment measures, such as the Geriatric Rating Scale (Kane & Kane, 1981; Plutchik et al. 1970) is needed for nursing assessment of demented patients. Using these instruments researchers must take into account the highly variable cognitive, psychosocial, and physical deficits among Alzheimer's disease patients and the interaction of these deficits with the patient's specific environment. The effect of cognitive function on performance of activities of daily living and the associated nursing interventions are two other critical issues that must be addressed by nursing research (Beck, 1988).

CLIENT RESPONSES AND NURSING INTERVENTIONS

Nursing interventions in Alzheimer's disease are specific compensations for an individual's deficits secondary to the disease process. Interventions are based on the individual's remaining capacities and are supportive rather than curative. Thus validation of the behavioral correlates at each stage of Alzheimer's disease are important for designing and testing nursing interventions.

Nursing studies of interventions are sparse and unintegrated. They are presented here in a settings-based framework (e.g., home-based or institutional care), as well as in the major categories of physical, emotional, cognitive/perceptual, and social care. Use of this framework indicates gaps in existing research and suggests possible avenues of fruitful inquiry.

Home-Based Care

Family Member Caregivers.   Studies of primary family caregivers of demented patients have shown that catastrophic reactions, waking at night, incontinence, suspiciousness, and communication were most problematic (Chenoweth & Spencer, 1986; Gmeiner, 1987; Rabins, Mace, & Lucas, 1982). Also identified as stressful were repetitive questions, communication issues, embarrassing behaviors, dangerous or hostile behavior, difficulty bathing, cooking, and providing care, incontinence, managing money, staying alone, caregiver stress, and lack of community support (Granow, 1988; Quayhagen & Quayhagen, 1988). Frequent night wakening, night wandering, and inability to drive a car safely, caregiver illness, inability of the caregiver to provide care, and hostile behavior were found to be significantly more frequent among patients who were subsequently institutionalized; and inability to find the bathroom, to recognize a spouse, to write, to drive, patient's depression, and occasional night waking and wandering were rated as more problematic by those who institutionalized their spouses (Chenoweth & Spencer, 1986; Gmeiner, 1987). The need to provide care was reported more frequently by those who institutionalized their Alzheimer's disease spouse. The more rapid the perceived rate of the patient's decline, the less verbal and more restless the patient, the older the spouse and the greater the fatigue of the spouse, the more apt the patient was to be institutionalized. These variables, along with ease of food preparation, predicted group membership (cared for at home or institutionalized) of 83% of the Alzheimer's disease patients studied.

Chenoweth and Spencer (1986) surveyed families of demented patients (N = 289, 45% homebound, 55% institutionalized) regarding recognition of the relative's cognitive problem, obtaining a diagnosis and assistive information, and reasons for institutionalization of the Alzheimer's disease relative. They found that the most common symptoms that prompted family members to seek medical assistance were: memory loss (52%) and problems related to personality changes, physical functional losses, work, driving, money management, and drinking (48%). Information given to family members at the time of diagnosis was: "nothing can be done, hopeless" (54%), factual, adequate explanation of Alzheimer's disease (28%), no information or explanation (20%), and advice for coping with behavioral problems or caregiving needs (16%). Family members generally reported that they sought and found a physician's advice helpful in deciding on institutionalization.

The basic social–psychological problem experienced by family caregivers in Wilson's (1989) qualitative study was confronting negative choices, defined as "different degrees of impossibility" and "undesirable alternatives" (p. 95). Caregivers have also reported that they had feelings of anger, depression, and fatigue (Rabins, Mace, & Lucas, 1982). However, in their intervention study of 19 family caregivers, Farran and Keane-Hagerty (1988) found that caregivers: (a) increased their repertoire of positive coping and problem-solving behaviors, and (b) increased reports of caregiving satisfaction after participating in a time-limited education support group. Thus, some family members of Alzheimer's disease patients, despite the difficulties of caregiving, can be assisted to increase coping and caregiving satisfaction. Farran and Keane-Hagerty also found that distress over memory problems increased significantly from pre- and postintervention measures.

Family members and clinicians tend to believe that behaviors before and after Alzheimer's disease are not related or connected. However, Shoemaker (1987), using retrospective interviews of family members to examine the behaviors of nine persons with Alzheimer's disease, found support for the hypothesis of continuity of comprehensible behavior. Four recurring themes were extracted from the data: hyperactivity, emotion, personal hygiene, and communication. Although behaviors and cognitive function varied after Alzheimer's disease, behavior was not as purposeless or unique as expected. Past behaviors tended to be more frequent and more intense, suggesting that Alzheimer's disease is not the sole explanation for all problematic behaviors.

Using controlled clinical trials, Chiverton and Caine (1989) investigated the effects of a brief educational program on the coping skills of spouses of patients with Alzheimer's disease who were living at home and examined whether the gender of the spouse affected coping abilities. Twenty spouses participated in an education program and were compared with 20 spouses who did not participate. Spouses who received the education felt significantly greater competence and functioned more independently, although some became distressed and overwhelmed with the information presented. No relationship between gender of spouse and coping ability was found.

Baldwin, Kleeman, Stevens, and Rasin (1989) randomly assigned caregivers who were caring for older persons with dementia to one of two treatment conditions (a didactic/educative and a support/psychotherapeutic program). The didactic/educative groups offered a classroom format with a defined curriculum focusing on family systems and family dynamics, stress and stress management, and differentiating normal from pathological aging. The support/psychotherapeutic group followed the form of a psychotherapy group, with topics and issues being introduced by the participants, with guidance, direction, and clarification by the co-leaders. Both the didactic/ educative and the support/psychotherapeutic groups were effective in reducing caregiver strain, with the support/psychotherapeutic group having the greatest and most lasting effect.

In a study of 10 family dyads (Alzheimer's disease patient and caregiver), Quayhagen and Quayhagen (1989) found that Alzheimer's disease patients maintained their levels of cognitive and behavioral functioning and improved emotionally following a home-based program of cognitive stimulation for both caregivers and the patients, whereas patients and caregivers who did not participate in the cognitive stimulation program did not improve. In this pilot study the researchers suggested that cognitive stimulation interventions hold promise for slowing the rate of cognitive decline in Alzheimer's disease patients if initiated in the early stages of the disease and deserve further nursing study. In addition, the cognitive stimulation program impacted positively on family members' well-being and enhanced their coping resources (Quayhagen & Quayhagen, 1989).

Work therapy for community-based Alzheimer's disease patients was studied by Ebbit, Burns, and Christensen (1989) and was found to be a potentially useful intervention for home-based patients and family members. Seven patients in the early and middle stages of Alzheimer's disease and their spouses participated in a sheltered work program two half days each week for 6 months. Work was supervised and tasks were adapted to the abilities of the Alzheimer's disease patients. All participants remained in the program throughout the study period. For six of the seven patients, depression scores decreased and self-esteem scores remained stable. Some anxiety was noted among both patients and family members, particularly at the beginning of the program. Mean family caregiver burden scores were also lower at the end of the 6 month program.

Problems discussed most frequently in support groups were lack of support and information from physicians, poor understanding of the disease, depression, a trapped feeling, anger and fear about the patient's behavior problems, social isolation, difficulties with role reversal, guilt about institutionalization of the Alzheimer's disease patient, and caregiver's loss of self-identity (Barnes, Raskind, Scott, & Murphy, 1981; Fruehwirth, 1989; Schmidt & Keyes, 1985). The major benefit reported was the discussion and sharing of information regarding caregiver problems. Schmidt and Keyes (1985) found that group members and leaders tended to avoid and stifle the free expression of feelings and concluded that the role of the leader is crucial.

Studies of support groups for husbands of Alzheimer's disease patients have been carried out by Moseley, Davies, and Priddy (1988). Bonding among the husbands for self help to deal with caregiver issues was described. The following themes were identified: (a) caregiver pride that motivated the husbands to action as a way of coping but often kept them from seeking needed assistance; (b) role changes that provided humor and less painful topics of discussion; (c) frustration and need for respite was acknowledged with older members of the group encouraging newer members to let go of guilt; (d) feelings were gradually expressed, although the men tended to avoid overt expression; and (e) caregiving was identified as an evolutionary process of becoming, assuming new roles, and beginning the grieving process. The investigators recommended that all male closed membership support groups have advantages for men who tend to be passive in the company of females and develop openness and trust slowly. They further suggested that reflective leader responses are more effective than confrontive or directive responses.

Respite Care.   Studies by nurses have examined the effects of respite programs. In a descriptive study, Miller, Gulle, and McCue (1986) evaluated two types of respite programs for family caregivers, a program for patients needing constant nursing attention and a residential program for patients requiring only housekeeping and companion services, in one New York suburban nursing home setting. Twenty two (22) respite participants were evaluated after one year of service. Staff reported that 13 of the respite clients appeared "reasonably content" during their stay. Seven family caregivers were enthusiastic, four were satisfied, and three were more open to long-term placement, however, four were dissatisfied. The researcher suggested that these four were dissatisfied because they were unable to give up caregiving control. Family caregivers also reported problems of excessive processing and cost for relatively short patient stays.

Using a pretest–posttest repeated measures design, the effects of a Day Away Centre on social and adaptive behaviors of elderly, geropsychiatric, mostly demented clients and on family caregiver stress was carried out by Johnson and Maguire (1989) in Australia. Findings included reductions in anxious and suspicious behaviors of clients, but no reduction in helplessness. Although family caregivers made positive remarks about the service, there was no significant decrease in stress scores. Additional nursing research on respite programs (e.g., adult day care, hospice care) is needed to assess the characteristics of Alzheimer's disease patients and families who use these services, the reasons respite programs are used or not used, the effects of specific programming on patients and family caregivers, and the costs of respite care.

Evaluation of Home-Based Care Research

Most of the studies of home-based care used small sample sizes ranging from 6 to 25 subjects (Barnes et al., 1981; Ebbitt et al., 1989; Farran & Keane-Hagerty, 1988; Fruehwirth, 1989; Granow, 1988; Johnson & Maguire, 1989; Miller et al., 1986; Moseley et al., 1988; Quayhagen & Quayhagen, 1989; Schmidt & Keyes, 1985; Shoemaker, 1987; Wilson, 1989; Sample sizes over 25 subjects were found in several studies (Baldwin et al., 1989; Chiverton & Caine, 1989; Evans et al., 1989; Gmeiner, 1987; Quayhagen & Quayhagen, 1988; Rabins et al., 1982), and one study reported a large sample size of 289 subjects (Chenoweth & Spencer, 1986). Most of the studies reported used descriptive or exploratory designs, content analysis and non parametric statistics for data analysis (Barnes et al., 1981; Chenoweth & Spencer, 1986; Evans, 1987; Farran & Keane-Hagerty, 1988; Fruehwirth, 1989; Gmeiner, 1987; Granow, 1988; Johnson, & Maguire, 1981; Miller et al., 1986; Moseley et al., 1988; Quayhagen & Quayhagen, 1988; Rabins et al., 1982; Schmidt & Keyes, 1985, Shoemaker, 1987; Wilson, 1989). Only a few researchers used a quasi-experimental design for their studies. Parametric statistics and tests of significance were used appropriately in these studies (Baldwin et al., 1989; Chiverton & Caine, 1989; Ebbitt et al., 1989; Quayhagen & Quayhagen, 1989) Because of the descriptive/exploratory nature of many studies, combined with small sample sizes, generalizability of the results is constrained.

Although nurse researchers are contributing substantially to the study of family caregivers of the dependent elderly (Archbold, 1983; Bowers, 1987; Given, King, Collins, & Given, 1988; Phillips & Rempusheski, 1986; Stommel, Given, & Given, 1990), fewer investigators have examined specifically family caregivers of Alzheimer's disease patients. In general, nursing research has emphasized the elder–caregiver relationship, caregiver feelings of stress and burden, and how nursing interventions can be provided. Additional research is needed to determine the extent to which findings regarding caregivers of dependent home-bound elders are generalizable to caregivers of Alzheimer's disease patients in the home. For example, the Beliefs about Caregiving Scale (BACS), that has been extensively tested by Phillips and her associates (Phillips & Rempusheski, 1986; Phillips, Rempusheski, & Morrison, 1989) with family caregivers of the frail elderly to identify caregivers who are at high risk for providing poor quality care to dependent elders at home should be evaluated with caregivers of Alzheimer's disease patients at home. Although the literature base on family caregivers of Alzheimer's disease patients is small, it indicates that nurse researchers are focusing on care problems and the meaning of the caregiving experience as defined by the caregivers.

Although a number of support group studies have been reported (e.g., Barnes et al., 1981; Davies, Priddy, & Tinklenberg, 1986; Fruehwirth, 1989; Moseley, Davies, & Priddy, 1988; Schmidt & Keyes, 1985), additional research is needed to evaluate the most effective leadership styles, group composition, and ways to facilitate access of family caregivers to support groups. Alternate ways of providing social support in the home and in the community through natural social networks also need investigation.

Review of nursing research on family caregivers at home indicates several methodological problems. For example, there is a lack of standardization of the meaning of caregiver, the level of caregiver needs tends to not be considered, most often only one family member caregiver is selected for study, most subjects are volunteers from self-help groups and may not be representative of caregivers in general, the Alzheimer's disease patients' perspectives regarding their care usually are not obtained (Barer & Johnson, 1990) and most studies have used a small number of subjects. Furthermore, most research has been focused on urban rather than rural caregivers and has primarily included white subjects, neglecting minority caregivers.

There is need to move beyond simple descriptive research of caregiver stress and its correlates. Multivariate models of caregiving should be tested with larger samples with clear criteria for the definition and inclusion of caregiver, multimethod approaches to measurement of the caregiving experience and evaluation of patterns of caregiving throughout the full duration of caregiving (Zarit, 1989a, 1989b). Controlled interventions studies are also essential. Nurse researchers should undertake the testing of interventions to make caregiving satisfying for Alzheimer's disease patients and families, such as in the study by Quayhagen and Quayhagen (1989). These studies should include measurement of the Alzheimer's disease patient's impairments and behaviors, the experiences of caregivers, and the desired outcomes of the intervention (Zarit, 1989a, 1989b).

There is a need for evaluation of respite care program effectiveness by nurses. Despite anecdotal evidence of the merits of respite and day care programs, there is little systematic evidence that these programs reduce caregiver stress or institutionalization of Alzheimer's disease patients. Nurse researchers need to better understand the objectives of respite and day care in order to study them. Cooperating relationships between researchers, clinicians, service providers, and funding agencies will advance this and other types of field research. For effective evaluation studies, demonstration and research must be coordinated from the outset so that baseline data can be systematically collected. Finally, control groups to strengthen the quasi-experimental designs that are more likely to be possible in field settings are essential for effective program evaluation.

Institutional Settings

Special Alzheimer's Care Units. Although the use of specially designed environments has been recognized as a needed intervention for persons with Alzheimer's disease, research to evaluate the effects on patients, families, staff caregivers, and cost has only been reported since the middle 1980s. Among the environmental interventions that have been proposed, Special Units (SUs) have been the most popular. Nursing homes often subscribe to the belief that SUs are effective in the care of Alzheimer's disease patients; most information that exists regarding cost effectiveness is anecdotal (Maas & Buckwalter, 1990).

There are several reports of nursing studies to evaluate the effects of SUs, however, most have not employed designs with sufficient control to rule out competing explanations (Cleary, Clamon, Price, & Shullaw, 1988; Greene, Asp, & Crane, 1985; Hall, Kirschling, & Todd, 1986; Matthew, Sloan, Kilby, & Flood, 1988). Research by Maas and Buckwalter (1990) using random assignment of Alzheimer's disease patients to experimental (SU) and control (traditional nursing units) groups and pre- and posttest repeated measures to assess the effects of the Special Units strategy, is an exception. For this study, Maas (1988) modified the Progressively Lowered Threshold model as a conceptual framework. Initial analysis revealed no significant changes in cognitive or functional abilities over time and no significant differences in these abilities between Alzheimer's disease patients on the Special Unit and on traditional integrated nursing home units. Patients on the Special Unit were restrained less than those living on traditional units, but the Special Unit patients fell significantly more, on the average. The total number of medications for each patient was not significantly different for Special Unit versus traditional unit patients and the number per patient did not increase over the one-year study period.

Matthew and associates (1988) studied 13 dementia patients in one Special Unit and 34 patients in two comparison settings; other wards in the nursing home with the Special Unit, and another nursing home. Data were collected from observations, existing clinical records, and clinical examinations. More Special Unit than comparison patients were private pay, had a specific diagnosis of Alzheimer's disease, had fewer additional medical diagnoses, less frequent use of physical restraints, and had families with high satisfaction with care. There was a trend toward more Special Unit patients being Caucasian, receiving more psychotropic medications, having more documented injuries and falls, and developing fewer decubiti. No differences were found in cognitive or functional status between the demented Special Unit patients and the comparison patients.

Behavioral characteristics of 6 Alzheimer's disease patients before and after care on a SU in a 180-bed nursing home were reported by Greene, Asp, and Crane (1985). An average of 43% of the patients had negative behaviors (e.g., hostile, agitated, incontinent, combative) reported while the patients were living on traditional units, compared to 3% of patients with negative behaviors while living on the Special Unit.

The effects of a Reduced Stimulation Unit (RSU) in a nonprofit life care center on patients, staff, and family members was evaluated by Cleary and colleagues (1988). A pretest–posttest design with multiple measures was used. All patients who were transferred to the Reduced Stimulation Unit had previously been cared for on the same traditional nursing care unit. Patients showed a significant improvement in performance of activities of daily living, but not in emotional and mental characteristics. There was a statistically significant increase in patients' average weight, a significant reduction in use of physical restraints, no change in sleep patterns, and no differences in the levels of tranquilizing medications. Significant improvement in family member satisfaction with care was noted, although family satisfaction was quite high prior to opening of the RSU. Staff knowledge and satisfaction did not change significantly from pretest to posttest. This study did not employ a control group and used a small number of subjects. Little description of the RSU was provided with no detail regarding the number and interval of repeated measurements nor much information regarding data analysis procedures used.

Hall and associates (1986) studied 12 Alzheimer's disease patients after they were moved to a Low Stimulus Unit in an 89-bed nursing home. Subjects were evaluated for 3 months following transfer to the unit. An increase in interaction and social support among the Alzheimer's disease patients, an increase in socialization at mealtime, and an increase in weight or decrease in weight loss for all but one patient, was observed. Prescription of tranquilizers decreased, all patients slept at night without sedation, a decrease in prn (as needed) sedation, and decreases in agitation, combative behavior, and wandering episodes also were noted.

The use of the Dementia Behavior Scale (Haycox, 1984) to screen patients for admission to a closed Alzheimer's disease unit was tested by

McCraken and Fitzwater (1989). After the scale had been in use for a year, initial and monthly follow-up assessments were compared for 11 Alzheimer's disease patients admitted to the unit. On admission, the patients functioned best in motor coordination and worst in dressing/grooming. At the end of the year, average scores had improved in all categories (language/conversation, social interaction, attention/ awareness, spatial orientation, motor coordination, bowel/bladder, eating/nutrition) except motor coordination and dressing/grooming. The authors concluded that this instrument is a useful screening tool for determination of placement of patients on SUs or traditional units.

Physical Component. Rheaume, Riley, and Volicer (1987) compared the energy intake (diet) and expenditure (weight, sleep, and miles paced per day) of three pacing and three nonpacing Alzheimer's disease patients. While duration of sleep was similar in both groups, the pacers expended 1600 kcal per day, a significant difference from the nonpacers. The researchers concluded that there were no significant weight losses in the pacing group because they had been placed on a special hypercaloric diet, however, these findings should be validated with a much larger group.

Sleep/wake cycles often are disrupted in the patient with Alzheimer's disease. Nursing research is needed to evaluate the effectiveness of daytime naps/rest periods on nighttime wakefulness, the relationship of sleep cycle disturbances to use of sedative-hypnotic and psychotropic medications, and environmental factors such as color of nurses' uniforms (Steffes & Thralow, 1985). Manipulation of rigid institutional schedules to reflect changing sleep patterns in the elderly also should be examined. Steffes and Thralow (1985) found that cognitively and visually impaired elderly subjects had increased disturbed behavior at night after nursing rounds conducted by nurses wearing white uniforms as compared to nurses in brown uniforms. Clapin-French (1986) found that patients were receiving large amounts of sleep medication although their nurses were assessing their sleep histories inaccurately, if at all. Thus, nurses were not comprehensively assessing factors that might be related to patients' insomnia.

Incontinence is common among long-term care (LTC) residents with Alzheimer's disease and may be caused by a variety of medical conditions, sensory perceptual deficiencies, and environmental factors. Feedback techniques have proved useful in retraining patients to interpret feelings of bladder fullness and deserve further attention. O'Donnell and Beck (1987) used a biofeedback technique that allowed the patient to relearn the feeling of bladder fullness so that they could contract their own sphincter to control urination. Clay (1978) attempted to reverse incontinence with four demented elderly subjects. Habit training was used with social and self-reinforcement. Two of the four patients improved, one was completely continent with reminders, and one did not improve. The effectiveness of reorientation and remotivation techniques (signs, color coding and other visual cues, behavioral training) also deserves further study.

Safety issues related to falls, elopement, physical aggression and re-straints are primary concerns in the care of demented individuals residing in long-term care facilities. In a study to describe falls and test falls precautions on a geropsychiatric unit, Hernandez and Miller (1986) studied 108 falls in the first year of a two-year period in a 21-bed geropsychiatric unit for persons over age 62 in a large care center/hospital. The sample consisted of 20 fallers and 56 nonfallers. Of the fallers, 71% had a diagnosis of depression, and 46% had a diagnosis of dementia, compared with 75% depressed and 10% de-mented nonfallers. They reported that investigations of the benefits of raising side rails to prevent falls were inconclusive. Patients with gait disorders and poor balance are at risk for falls and apraxia is the gait most commonly associated with the later stages of Alzheimer's disease.

Emotional Component.   Mayers and Griffin (1990) studied the re-sponses of demented patients to a variety of toys and stimulus objects. Five severely impaired Alzheimer's disease patients and 4 patients with dementia secondary to alcohol abuse were provided with 10 separate stimulus items (e.g., plush toy, keys, small metal cars) over the course of a 2-week period. The same objects were presented to the Alzheimer's disease patients in the same manner 3 months later. Most interest was displayed in stimulus objects appropriate for infants and preschoolers, such as toys that had movable parts, although the patients also showed considerable interest in plush toys and dolls. The investigators' impression was that the patients were more calm after exploration of the toys. They caution that use of stimulus objects must be shaped to individual needs and cognitive abilities and that further research is needed to test areas of environmental control over agitation and stimulus enhancement.

Cognitive/Perceptual Component.   Many components of cognition are altered with the progression of Alzheimer's disease. For example, perceptual deficits and the inability to recognize and correctly interpret objects in the environment have a profound effect on nursing care. Distorted perceptions often lead to psychiatric symptoms such as illusions, delusions, and pseudo-hallucinations that are disturbing to both patients and staff. Apraxia and other motor behaviors interfere with Alzheimer's disease victims' ability to perform activities of daily living. Falls and wandering are behaviors that pose very difficult care problems for nurses.

Norberg, Melvin, and Asplund (1986) explored the reactions of two patients in the final stages of Alzheimer's disease. Each patient received 16 trials of a standardized sequence of music, touch, and object presentation stimulation during 12 consecutive days. Evaluations were by direct observation, analysis of videotaped recordings, and measurement of pulse and respiration rates. After stimulating the patients with music, touch, and object presentations, their motor behavior and vital signs were analyzed. Both patients reacted differently to music than to touch and object presentation with change in pulse in response to a specific tune noted for each patient. Because only two patients were used and each had a unique behavioral response, different variables were estimated for each and each served as his own control.

Using a 12-step classification system with 5 patients in different stages of Alzheimer's disease, Sandman et al. (1986) quantitatively assessed self-care capability. Subjects were able to care for themselves independently and there was wide variation in performance from day to day. Apraxia was a crucial factor in determining ability, as were paratonia and motivation to a lesser degree. Verbal and nonverbal directions only marginally influenced the level of apraxia. The researchers concluded that the patients' highest level of performance was primarily dependent on the patient–nurse interaction. A primary example of effective patient–nurse interaction is assistance in initiating tasks (e.g., giving the client soap, washcloth, and water rather than telling the client to wash).

Orientation and memory problems are among the earliest problems encountered with Alzheimer's disease. Nursing strategies such as cueing, prompting, visual imagery, stress-reduction, and reinforcement also deserve further evaluation. An experimental pilot study of the effects of cognitive skills remediation training on the areas of attention and reading, remembering and concentrating on details was carried out by Beck, Heacock, Mercer, Thatcher, and Sparkman (1988). Areas of cognitive function were tested before and after the cognitive skills training and the results compared to data from a control group that received no intervention. No significant differences between the two groups were found. However, when change scores were compared, there was a statistically significant difference for recalling numbers on a list, a remembering function that may have important implications for the ability to carry out activities of daily living. Because of the pilot nature of the study, small sample size, and the fact that subjects were not matched for sex, living arrangements, and marital status, the authors note that interpretation must be made cautiously. Because pre- and posttest cognitive skills test scores were so close, there was little room for detection of differences between the groups.

Rosswurm (1989) compared 30 Alzheimer's disease patients' and 30 nondemented older adults' performances on visual matching tasks to assess sensory detection, attention, recognition, and short-term recall. The Alzheimer's disease patients had more difficulty with matching patterns than with single dimension stimuli. As expected, poorest performance of Alzheimer's disease patients occurred with recall tasks, supporting the hypothesis that perceptual processing deficits in early stages of information acquisition contribute to memory problems. Alzheimer's disease patients also improved their recall performance 90% when given verbal encoding cues. Nondemented elders had minimal difficulty with all tasks and improved recall 100% with encoding. According to Rosswurm (1989), the findings provide evidence of perceptual deficits in Alzheimer's disease patients during obtaining information and suggest that nurses should study the effectiveness of limiting the number of items of information and distractors in the environment, using encoding and providing verbal descriptions of stimuli. The investigator further suggested the need for a longitudinal study of persons in the early stage of Alzheimer's disease to gather data on changes in processing deficits as the disease progresses.

Reality Orientation.   Reality Orientation has received very little empirical support as an effective mechanism for reducing confusion and disorientation, especially over time. Several nurse researchers have questioned the value of reality orientation with demented patients (Akerlund & Norberg, 1986; Ricci, 1983; Schwab, Rader, & Doan, 1985). Akerlund and Norberg (1986) compared the effects of reality orientation and psychotherapy on the mental status of demented patients in a psychogeriatric clinic ward in Sweden and provided evidence that the patients were more active and their conversation was on a higher cognitive level during psychotherapy sessions than in the reality orientation group. Using observation and critique of video tapes, the investigators subsequently conducted a pilot study of psychotherapy with four demented patients and noted that "the most striking difference between the reality–orientation group and the psychodynamic pilot group was the amount of verbal activity by several demented patients" (p. 84). The researchers concluded that more dynamic approaches need to be developed and tested to improve demented patients' behavior.

Validation Therapy.   Validation therapy (Feil, 1982), an alternative to reality orientation that does not aim to increase awareness of reality, was studied by Robb, Stegman, and Wolanin (1986). Using an experimental design, 16 dementia patients were randomly assigned to a control group and 20 assigned to an experimental group. A twice weekly validation therapy program was implemented for 9 months with experimental subjects. Data were analyzed for 12 control, 9 experimental, and 6 subjects who were randomly assigned to the experimental group, but did not attend a majority of the therapy meetings. No statistically significant differences in mental status, morale, and social behavior were found on pre- and posttest measures for any of the three groups or between posttest measures for experimental and control groups.

Wandering.   Wandering is a care problem for which nursing research efforts are beginning to have considerable clinical impact in guiding nursing interventions, although much remains to be understood about wanderers and their behavior. Rosswurm, Zimmerman, Schwartz-Fulton, and Norman (1986) investigated the wandering behavior of nine nursing home residents with Alzheimer's disease. The descriptive analysis of observations of location, activity, and interaction revealed wandering patterns that were amendable to controlled environmental stimuli (activity-dining room, large photos of residents by their bedroom doors) and planned group activities (group walks, exercises, dances, rhythm instrument playing, beach ball games, and pet therapy). Postintervention observations included more frequent wandering in the activity-dining area and less frequent wandering in other residents' rooms, decreased daytime sleeping and nonpurposeful hand movements, and an increase in walking as opposed to sitting. Unexpected findings were increased group identification and increased positive response to others during group activities. The investigators emphasized the need for further study of Alzheimer's disease residents' responses to group identity.

In Shoemaker's (1987) study of wanderers using observation of patients and reactions of family members, hyperactivity, emotion, personal hygiene, and communication were recurring themes. Wandering was not observed or reported for all patients and when it was observed, it was not purposeless. Premorbid factors seemed to be related to the propensity to wander. That is, wandering was associated with some premorbid lifestyle factor such as work or shopping. Thus, this study provided some evidence to support Snyder, Rupprecht, Pyret, Brekhus, and Moss' (1978) hypothesis that wandering is related to premorbid psychosocial factors, and also the early work of Monsour and Robb (1982) who identified wandering as consistent with lifelong behavior patterns.

Nocturnal wandering was studied in 8 (4 male, 4 female) elderly Alzheimer's patients on a hospital gerontological research unit to evaluate the use of "modified white noise" (Young, Muir-Nash, & Ninos, 1988). White noise is defined as any low intensity, slow, continuous, rhythmic, monotonous sound, for example the whir of a fan or the hum of an air conditioner. Subjects were randomly assigned to 2 groups and followed for 12 nights. Repeated measures analysis of variance showed no significant effects due to treatment or group. However, when subjects were analyzed individually, significant decreases in agitated and restless behavior were found for two patients during the treatment phase.

Social Component. Nursing studies of institutionalized demented patients have been focused primarily on the environment, social interaction, aggressive behavior, and caregiver stress. Caregiver stress is addressed elsewhere in this review. More research is needed to evaluate the effects of enhancing Alzheimer's disease patients' sense of mastery and control over the environment. More rigorous nursing research is needed in the area of nonverbal communication abilities, focusing on touch, facial expression, eye contact, tone of voice, and posture. In this regard group therapy approaches and use of plush animals (Francis & Baly, 1986) should be tested with Alzheimer's disease subjects. Research by Beck (1982) suggested that approaches designed to stimulate awareness and control of surroundings also increase cognitive activity among nursing home residents. Research on methods to enhance social interaction and social skills in institutionalized residents with Alzheimer's disease is needed.

Ryden (1988) studied aggressive behaviors of 124 patients in 4 nursing homes using the Ryden Aggression Scale Form 2 (RAS). The RAS is a 25-item instrument using a Likert-type rating scale. The three subscales include physical, verbal, and sexual aggressive behavior. Content validity was reported. Test–retest reliability was .86; internal consistency (Cronbach's alpha) coefficient were: .88 (overall), .84 (physical aggression), .90 (verbal aggression), and .74 (sexual aggression). Some form of aggression was found in 66% of patients. Neither degree of cognitive impairment nor extent of physical dependency was associated with aggression. The majority of incidents of aggression were in response to touch or invasion of personal space and occurred on the day shift. Meddaugh (1991) conducted a qualitative, exploratory investigation examining the similarities and differences between 27 aggressive and nonaggressive demented patients. Past life experiences, rather than personality characteristics or degree of cognitive impairment, impacted on acclimation to a new environment.

Nurses must alter normal communication patterns to compensate for language losses associated with Alzheimer's disease. Langland and Panicucci (1982) found an increase in facial expression, eye contact, and body movements in confused elderly patients with whom touch was used with verbal requests. Similarly, Burnside (1979) noted subjective improvement in six regressed clients with whom touch was used.

The effects of the use of a pet dog as a therapeutic agent for persons residing in a Special Alzheimer's Care Unit were assessed by Kongable, Buckwalter, and Stolley (1989). Social behaviors of the Alzheimer's disease patients during the permanent residence of the therapy dog, during temporary visits by the dog, and when the dog was absent, were compared. Social behaviors also were compared for periods when the dog visited patients individually and when the dog visited the same patients in a group. The results from a repeated measures within subject design analysis revealed a significantly greater number of social behaviors ($p < 0.001$) when the dog was in permanent residence and when the dog visited the Alzheimer's disease patients individually.

Family Members of Institutionalized Alzheimer's Disease Patient. In a repeated measures descriptive study of 38 family members, Maas, Buckwalter and Kelley (in press) found that most family members continued to visit on a regular basis and were moderately to highly satisfied with the care of their Alzheimer's disease relatives in a long-term care facility. However, the family members' perceptions of care, as measured by the Family Perceptions Tool (FPT) was developed by the investigators. Test–retest reliability of the FPT ranged from .78 to .90 ($p < .05$). Content validity was established by a panel of gerontological nurses and social workers who reviewed and revised the instrument. Cronbach's alpha coefficients for the four subscales were .77 to .87 (satisfaction with environment), .91 to .93 (satisfaction with physical care), .74 to .92 (satisfaction with staff relationships), and .91 to .93 (satisfaction with overall care). Results indicated that families were less satisfied with nursing care than with care provided by other health disciplines. Family members also had the most frequent contact with nurses, which may create more opportunities for role conflicts, ambiguities, and incongruities than with members of other disciplines. The investigators reasoned that diminished satisfaction with care by nurses was likely because of family feelings associated with the transition from primary caregivers with high control over care priorities to visitor status with low control. Family members also were consistently least satisfied with resources available for the care of their relatives with Alzheimer's disease throughout the 12 month study period. This finding may be a result of the low level of funding for long-term care by state and federal government and small proportion of professional compared to nonprofessional caregiver staff that are typical of most long-term care facilities.

Staff Caregivers. Nursing studies of staff caregivers of Alzheimer's disease patients is another neglected area of research. Norberg and colleagues (Akerlund & Norberg, 1985; Norberg, Asplund, & Waxman, 1987; Bexell, Norberg, & Norberg, 1985; Norberg & Hirschfeld, 1987; Norberg & Asplund, 1990) have explored the meaning to staff of feeding severely demented patients. Ethical models associated with their reasoning were also examined. Their research has shown that in feeding the severely demented, staff are sometimes uncertain that they are helping the patient (Akerlund & Norberg, 1985; Norberg, Asplund, & Waxman, 1987). Using a teleological ethical model, an activity is meaningful if: (a) it has intrinsic merit, (b) it is not pointless, (c) it has sufficient worth, (d) its worthy end is achievable at reasonable cost (Joske, 1974). In Israel, many staff caregivers were found to not question their feeding of severely demented patients because they thought of it as their duty, based on the principle of sanctity of life (Norberg & Hirschfeld, 1987). Most Swedish caregivers discussed meaning for the patient from the perspective of the patient's experience rather than intrinsic meaning. They reported relief when the patient died and was spared from further suffering and felt that caregiving was satisfying because of caring and being helpful (Norberg & Asplund, 1990). That contact with the demented patient can provide meaning is a consistent finding with a previous study (Akerlund & Norberg, 1990). Additional findings were that being able to help the patient also gave meaning to caregiving, based on a value of interdependence; the more helpless the demented patient, the greater the feeling of responsibility and duty and the more the caregivers' own needs were met (Norberg & Asplund, 1990).

Gillis, Whall, Booth, and Beel-Bates (1989) described the most difficult to manage disruptive behaviors of elderly patients in nursing homes and nursing strategies used to manage these behaviors from the perspective of nursing staff. One hundred forty seven nursing staff in 14 nursing homes participated in the survey. No significant differences were found in disruptive behaviors or management strategies as reported by licensed and nonlicensed nursing staff. More than three fourths of the elderly who were reported by the nursing staff as disruptive were also cognitively impaired. The management strategies reported by the staff included verbal discussion (66%), followed by chemical restraints (50%) and physical restraints (43%). However, 40% of staff also reported using time-out and 23% reported using activity diversion, indicating staff knowledge of some forms of behavior modification.

Maas and Buckwalter (1990) included analysis of effects on staff knowledge, caregiver stress, burnout, job satisfaction, turnover, and absenteeism in their evaluation study of a Special Alzheimers Unit. Preliminary findings indicated that scores for RN staff knowledge about Alzheimer's disease were consistently higher throughout the study than non RN nursing staff knowledge scores. RNs working on the Special Unit were significantly more satisfied with their preparation than were other nursing staff, whether they were on the Special Unit or traditional units. Overall, all staff were moderately highly satisfied with their work throughout the study period. Nursing staff on the Special Unit experienced a significant reduction in stress, while control nursing staff stress increased over time. The staff on the Special Unit with reduced stress tended to be more senior. Nursing staff on the Special Unit had significantly less burnout than staff on traditional units. Finally, RNs on the Special Unit had a significant decrease in the use of sick time, while non RN nursing staff use of sick time did not change significantly.

In a qualitative study of staff responses to the presence of a therapy dog on a Special Unit for Alzheimer's clients, Kongable, Stolley, and Buckwalter (1990) reported positive responses by staff for pet therapy. Staff expressed a sense of enthusiasm and commitment toward the pet therapy program, and expressed concern for client safety (therapy dog becoming aggressive or causing falls), safety of the dog (clients becoming aggressive toward the dog), and administrative issues (budget, care of the dog, etc.).

Cost of Care. Considerable costs are involved in the care of Alzheimer's disease patients in nursing homes and interventions are often implemented without systematic testing of their cost effectiveness. There is agreement that quality care requires changes in the physical environment, more staffing, and better trained staff (OTA, 1987). Special Care Units, however, have proliferated without rigorous evaluation, including a comparison of costs of care on Special Units and traditional, integrated units. Although results have not yet been reported, the Maas and Buckwalter (1990) nursing evaluation research of a Special Unit was the only nursing study located that included cost as an effect variable.

EVALUATION OF RESEARCH IN INSTITUTIONS

Nursing research of Special Units (SU) has been largely nonsystematic. Researchers have not included a description of the characteristics of the Special Unit, have not used a control or comparison group and have tended to provide little or no description of how variables were measured. Definition of what a good "SU" is and detailed descriptions of SUs are lacking. As Ohta and Ohta (1988) noted in a recent overview of SU research, nursing studies suffer from a lack of specification and standardization of Special Unit characteristics (philosophy, environmental design, therapeutic programming, staffing, staff training, patient admission, and discharge criteria), the use of nonexperimental designs, and measurement tools that are inappropriate for the population studied, and that lack adequate psychometric evaluation. Some Alzheimer's disease patients may function best on open, traditional units, especially in the early stages of the disease. Those in the late stage of the disease require skilled nursing care. There is a need to test a taxonomy of SU characteristics on a range of cognitively impaired patients, their family members and staff caregivers, and to evaluate cost factors associated with SUs. The development and testing of reliable and valid tools to guide placement of Alzheimer's disease residents is needed also. Implementation of state and national registries of SUs, including detailed documentation of philosophy, environmental design, programming, staffing, staff training, and patient admission and discharge criteria are needed in order to develop a taxonomy of Special Units so that the effects of different types of SUs could be tested on patients, families, and staff caregivers.

More research is needed on the many aspects of care of Alzheimer's disease patients. A few studies have been done by nurses on sleep, bladder function, nutrition, wandering, and safety. Research to describe specific care problems of Alzheimer's disease patients is essential so that interventions for their management, particularly oral hygiene maintenance, swallowing, nutrition, and prevention of protein calorie malnutrition in this population can be developed and tested.

There is a paucity of research-based interventions related to the idiosyncratic and often exaggerated emotional responses associated with Alzheimer's disease. Beck and Heacock (1988) have identified a number of areas for nursing interventions and research, including sexual behavior, anxiety, catastrophic reactions, and depression. Aberrant sexual behavior may occur in Alzheimer's disease because of impaired inhibitions and judgment. Nursing research is needed to understand the circumstances of hypersexual behavior and to test interventions for patients, family members, and staff caregivers.

Research is also needed to determine the effectiveness of nursing interventions (such as simplification of routines, information giving and choices, exercise, and relaxation techniques) in the management of anxiety in patients with Alzheimer's disease. Prevention and management of catastrophic reactions is another fertile area for nursing research. Particular attention should be paid to the development and testing of interventions, such as diversionary tactics, that deal with angry and aggressive behaviors. It is known that depression and anxiety can contribute to excess disability. Researchers should examine the use of scales that measure these emotional components and determine their reliability and validity in persons with Alzheimer's disease. Researchers should also investigate the effect of emotional disorders on the cognitive and functional abilities of persons with Alzheimer's disease.

More testing of environmental modifications, behavioral techniques, sequencing, and cueing mechanisms to reduce cognitive and perceptual difficulties is sorely needed. Research on the benefits of cognitive retraining, cognitive restructuring, and cognitive remediation techniques on short-term memory is equivocal and worthy of more study. Feil's (1982) concept of validation therapy requires further rigorous research, as does the psychodynamic group approach described by Akerlund and Norberg (1986).

Research efforts such as those described earlier help nurses conceptualize wandering behavior and should lead to additional studies to evaluate the effects of nursing interventions on wandering. Technological methods, more sensitive than the pedometer, to assess wandering are needed. More research is also needed on falls prevention in this population, since the fear of patient falls and injuries promotes the use of physical and/or chemical restraints. The relationships of falls, particularly injurious falls, to cognitive status, functional status, morbidity of other illnesses, and specific types of treatments and medications deserve further study. Because hostile, aggressive behavior and communication difficulties are frequently cited as problems for caregivers, further research should be conducted on these problems as well.

More nursing research is needed to assess the effects of pet therapy, including the benefits of various kinds of pets and different models of pet management along the continuum of care. Other interventions on Alzheimer's disease patients' social behaviors also require systematic testing. Particular attention should be given to distinguishing the characteristics of patients who benefit most from particular interventions and the cost effectiveness of interventions as well as staff perceptions.

There is a paucity of research regarding family members following institutionalization of their Alzheimer's disease relatives. Yet, as Wilson (1989) found in her study of family caregivers, institutionalization "is a dreaded eventuality and the decision poses the ultimate negative choice for caregivers" (p. 98). Research is needed to document the needs and resources of family members, the sources of satisfaction and dissatisfaction with the care of patients, and the effectiveness of alternative nursing interventions to facilitate family member role transition and continued participation in the patients' care following institutionalization (Maas, Buckwalter, & Kelley, 1991). Development and testing of instruments to measure family members' satisfaction with care and with their roles when their Alzheimer's disease relatives are in an institution should have priority.

No published studies of stress, job satisfaction, or knowledge and understanding of Alzheimer's disease were located except those reported by Cleary and associates (1988) and Maas and Buckwalter (1990). These are clearly neglected and important areas of nursing research as Alzheimer's disease patients have been estimated to comprise as much as 65% of persons in nursing homes and the management of these behaviors presents many difficult and costly care problems (Hing, 1987).

RESEARCH ISSUES

Methodological Issues

A number of methodological issues related to research with the elderly noted by Gueldner and Hanner (1989) are relevant to nursing research in Alzheimer's disease. First, it is difficult, if not impossible, to obtain representative samples because there often are no centralized lists that can be released. Alzheimer's disease patients are quite varied although they are often treated as a homogeneous group. It is therefore important that researchers specify the demographic and functional characteristics of subjects and study related behavioral differences.

Recruitment of Alzheimer's disease family subjects can be problematic as family caregivers are often frail, may be reluctant to participate in research, and are fearful of signing any papers. Person-to-person contact is usually most effective but very time-consuming. Special care must be taken with informed consent procedures for Alzheimer's disease patients because of cognitive impairment. For many persons with Alzheimer's disease, a legal guardian or a relative may be required to sign a consent form. As many as 46% of relatives of nursing home residents have refused to allow research participation when approached (Warren et al., 1986). Moreover, written descriptions of risks of the research can reinforce, rather than reduce fears of elderly persons or their legal representatives. If the person with Alzheimer's disease is living in a nursing home, the assistance of trusted staff is apt to be necessary.

The reliability and validity of many existing measurement tools cannot be assumed and there is a need to establish psychometric properties with Alzheimer's disease patient and caregiver populations. Special attention should be given to presentation of response options for elderly subjects and family members because of the possibility of cognitive and perceptual problems. Educational level of some age cohorts of patients and families also may be related to specific response patterns and to abilities to interpret questions and supply valid responses. Physical disabilities due to illnesses such as arthritis or stroke also can make responding to written questionnaires difficult. Anxieties, fears, and some attitudes of the elderly can be adversely affected by questionnaire or interview items if not carefully phrased, making the data of questionable validity. The elderly often are sensitive about questions regarding income. Finally, instruments that require more than 25 minutes to administer are likely to not be completed by a substantial percentage of the elderly. As a solution to many of these methodological problems, some nurse researchers favor an interview approach with all elderly subjects. While this approach is costly in terms of research staff time, the opportunity to ascertain and correct misinterpretation of questions is enhanced.

Nursing research with Alzheimer's disease patients must deal with these methodological issues related to the elderly in general, as well as additional problems specific to persons with Alzheimer's disease. Studies that seek to test specific nursing interventions in institutions often must be content with small numbers of subjects or use multiple sites. Thus, studies can yield less than 20 subjects, especially if longitudinal data are required, largely due to attrition from death. The rigor of designs that can be used and the power of statistical tests to detect differences is greatly reduced with these small sample sizes. The use of multiple sites to increase the number of subjects is very costly in terms of staff time and dollars, making extramural funding more difficult to obtain.

A number of problems of control that are characteristic of field research in general and that threaten the integrity of rigorous, systematic research also are troublesome for nurse researchers in Alzheimer's disease. Compromises to the internal and external validity of field experiments should be made explicit and the results should be discussed in terms of these limitations in research reports. The lack of a definitive diagnosis, except at autopsy, makes it likely that some research labeled as Alzheimer's disease studies actually includes patients with other irreversible dementias. While from a behavioral management perspective the specific type of dementia would not appear to be an important variable, the differences in manifestations of the diseases and the efficacies of interventions for each are not fully known and require closer examination.

The dependence on clinical staff for cooperation and assistance with research on Alzheimer's disease patients has several disadvantages. For example, staff may resent the intrusion on their time and energies. This is a difficult problem because most nursing homes are short of staff and other resources. There is also the danger that the research will be obtrusive and alter the nature of the treatment that is being studied. In field research, control of the treatment variable and of completing plausible explanations for findings are often compromised. As noted earlier, Alzheimer's disease patients and their caregivers are not homogeneous groups. Thus, replication of studies in multiple settings with multiple populations is necessary to generate a nursing knowledge base in this area.

RECOMMENDATIONS FOR FUTURE NURSING RESEARCH ON ALZHEIMER'S DISEASE

Recommendations for promising areas of nursing research include the identification of functional strengths of Alzheimer's disease patients (physical, cognitive, emotional, social/behavioral) that can serve as the basis for treatment and the management of specific behavioral problems (e.g., agitated behavior, catastrophic reactions, hallucinations/paranoia, incontinence, wandering). Research also is needed to test physical cues in the environment, social cues to reinforce the meaning of physical cues, and continuity of person and daily routine in reducing and adjusting disordered person-environment interaction (Roberts & Algase, 1988). Studies to examine treatment modalities relevant to the cognitive/perceptual, emotional, social/behavioral, and physical problems associated with Alzheimer's disease, focusing attention on the efficacy of different modalities to reduce excess disability in the Alzheimer's disease patient and to reduce family and staff caregiver stress, should be carried out. Identification and testing of interventions to alleviate reversible physical and emotional disabilities in Alzheimer's disease patients also are needed. Cognitive skills assessment and remediation warrant further investigation to determine if certain subgroups of Alzheimer's disease patients benefit most from specific interventions. Modification of the interpersonal and/or physical environment of Alzheimer's disease patients in long-term care facilities, including cost measurements, are additional areas to address. Replication of isolated studies with different subjects and situations are encouraged to increase confidence in the generalizability of results.

The development of appropriate, effective, and safe services for the care and support of Alzheimer's disease patients and their families in the home, in long-term care, and in other settings is a particular challenge. More needs to be known about what patient behaviors are associated with what types and what levels of caregiver burden and stress. Interventions should be designed to be congruent with the needs of family caregivers and evaluated according to caregivers' perceived benefits. Whether family members have appropriate roles in collaborative staff-family efforts also needs to be examined (Buckwalter & Hall, 1987). Little is known about the positive experiences of caregiving, if any. More needs to be known about the types of care provided by family caregivers and the knowledge needed to provide these services over time without undue burden. The effects of family involvement in nursing homes in an adjunct staff capacity (e.g., as co-group leaders of remotivation, movement, and music groups) should be explored. Cross cultural nursing research that examines the characteristics and behaviors of Alzheimer's disease patients and family caregivers and the efficacy of nursing interventions to alleviate dysfunction in minority populations are another priority.

Nursing research on what level of staff can carry out interventions effectively with Alzheimer's disease patients and families, the knowledge and training needed by all levels of nursing staff who care for Alzheimer's disease patients in the home and in institutions, and the effectiveness of different training approaches also is needed. Finally, there is need for study of ethical issues related to caring for Alzheimer's disease patients, especially the conflict between self-determination of the cognitively impaired and the provision of care that is of most benefit to the patient in the nurse's judgment.

SUMMARY

This chapter has included a review of nursing research in Alzheimer's disease. Much of what is in the literature regarding nursing of Alzheimer's disease patients and their families is anecdotal and has not been validated by systematic research and is atheoretical. The majority of nursing research on Alzheimer's disease has been focused on patient characteristics and problem behaviors or on the needs and experiences of family caregivers. Research should continue in these areas along with testing nursing interventions to maintain optimal cognitive, physical, social, and emotional function of Alzheimer's disease patients. Explanatory theories should be devised and tested to advance the development of nursing knowledge in the care of Alzheimer's disease patients and family caregivers. Finally, more evaluation research is needed to test the cost effectiveness of home-based and institutional programs, including effects on Alzheimer's disease patients, family members, and staff caregivers.

REFERENCES

Akerlund, B. M., & Norberg, A. (1985). An ethical analysis of double bind conflicts as experienced by care workers feeding severely demented patients. *International Journal of Nursing Studies, 22*, 207–216.

Akerlund, B. M., & Norberg, A. (1986). Group psychotherapy with demented patients. *Geriatric Nursing, 6*, 83–84.

Akerlund, B. M., & Norberg, A. (1990). Powerlessness in terminal care of demented patients: An exploratory study. *Omega, Journal of Death and Dying, 21*, 15–19.

Archbold, P. G. (1983). Impact of parent caring on middle-aged offspring. *Journal of Gerontological Nursing, 6*, 67–85.

Baldwin, B., Kleeman, K., Stevens, G., & Rasin, J. (1989). Family caregiver stress: Clinical assessment and management. *International Psychogeriatrics, 1*, 185–194.

Barer, B. M., & Johnson, C. L. (1990). A critique of the caregiving literature. *The Gerontologist, 30*, 26–29.

Barnes, R. F., Raskind M. A., Scott, M. A., & Murphy C. (1981). Problems of families caring for Alzheimer's patients: Use of a support group. *Journal of the American Geriatrics Society, 29*(2), 80–85.

Batt, L. J. (1989). Managing delirium: Implications for geropsychiatric nursing. *Journal of Psychosocial Nursing and Mental Health Service, 27*(5), 22–25.

Beck, P. (1982). Two successful interventions in nursing homes: The therapeutic effects of cognitive activity. *The Gerontologist, 22*, 378.

Beck, C. (1988). Measurement of dressing performance in persons with dementia. *The American Journal of Alzheimer's Care and Related Disorders & Research, 3*,(2), 21–25.

Beck, C., & Heacock, P. (1988). Nursing Interventions for patients with Alzheimer's disease. *Nursing Clinics of North America, 23*(1), 95–124.

Beck, C., Heacock, P., Mercer, S., Thatcher, R., & Sparkman, C. (1988). The impact of cognitive skills remediation training on persons with Alzheimer's disease or mixed dementia. *Journal of Geriatric Psychiatry, 11*(1), 773–788.

Bexell, G., Norberg, A., & Norberg, B. (1985). Ethical conflicts in long-term care of aged patients: An ontological model of the care situation. *Ethics and Medicine, 1*(3), 44–46.

Blass J. P. (1982). Dementia. *Medical Clinics of North America, 66*, 1143–1160.

Blass, J. P. (1990). The report of the advisory panel on Alzheimer's disease 1988–1989. *Generations, 14*(2), 68–69.

Booth, D., Bradley, W., & Whall, A. (1988). Description of early and late functional changes in persons with Alzheimer's disease, *Journal of Nursing Science and Practice, 1*(3), 9–16.

Bowers, B. J. (1987). Intergenerational caregiving: Adult caregivers and their aging parents. *Advances in Nursing Science, 9,*(2), 20–31.

Buckwalter, K. C., & Hall, G. R. (1987). Families of the institutionalized older adult: A neglected resource. In T. H. Brubaker (Ed.), *Aging, health, and families.* Newbury Park, CA: Sage Publications.

Burnside, I. M. (1979). Alzheimer's disease: An overview. *Journal of Gerontological Nursing, 5*(4), 14–20.

Campbell, E. B., Williams, M. A., & Mlynarczyk, S. M. (1986). After the fall. *American Journal of Nursing, 86,* 151–154.

Chenoweth, B., & Spencer, B. (1986). Dementia: The experience of family caregivers. *The Gerontologist, 26,* 267–272.

Chisholm S. E., Deniston, O. L., Igrisam, R. M., & Barbus A. J. (1982). Prevalence of confusion in elderly hospitalized patients. *Journal of Gerontological Nursing, 8*(2), 87–96.

Chiverton P., & Caine, E. D. (1989). Education to assist spouses coping with Alzheimer's disease: A controlled trial. *Journal of the American Geriatric Society, 37,* 593–598.

Clapin-French, E. (1986). Sleep patterns of aged persons in long-term care facilities. *Journal of Advanced Nursing, 11,* 57–66.

Clay, E. C. (1978). Incontinence of urine: A regime for retraining. *Nursing Mirror, 146,* 23–24.

Cleary, T. A., Clamon, C., Price, M., & Shullaw, G. (1988). A reduced stimulation unit: Effects on patients with Alzheimer's disease and related disorders. *The Gerontologist, 28,* 511–514.

Cohen, D., Kennedy, G., & Eisdorfer, C. (1984). Phases of changes in the patient with Alzheimer's dementia: A conceptual dimension for defining health care management. *Journal of the American Geriatrics Society, 32*(1), 11–15.

Cross, P. S., & Gurland, B. J. (1986). The epidemiology of dementing disorders. Contract report prepared for the Office of Technology Assessment, U.S. House of Representatives. Washington, DC: U.S. Government Printing Office.

Davies, H., Priddy, J. M., & Tinklerberg, J. (1986). Support groups for male caregivers of Alzheimer's patients. In Brink, T. J. (Ed.), *Clinical gerontology: A guide to assessment and intervention.* New York: The Haworth Press.

DeLong, A. (1970). The microspatial structure of the older person. In L. A. Pastalan & D. H. Carson (Eds.), *The spatial behavior of older people* (pp. 68–87). Ann Arbor, MI: University of Michigan Press.

Dennis, K. E., & Prescott, P. A. (1985). Florence Nightingale: Yesterday, today, and tomorrow. *Advances in Nursing Science, 7*(2), 66–81.

Doyle, G. C., Dunn, S., Thadani, I., & Lenihan, P. (1986). Investigating tools to aid in restorative care for Alzheimer's patients. *Journal of Gerontological Nursing, 12*(9), 19–24.

Ebbitt, B., Burns, T., & Christensen R. (1989). Work therapy: Intervention for community-based Alzheimer's patients. *American Journal of Alzheimer's Care and Related Disorders, 4*(5), 7–15.

Evans, L. K. (1987). Sundown Syndrome in institutionalized elderly. *Journal of the American Geriatrics Society, 35,* 101–108.

Evans, D. A., Funckenstein, H. H., Albert, M. S., Scherr, P. A., Cook, N. R., Chown, M. J., Hebert, L. E., Hennekens, C. H., & Taylor, J. O. (1989). Prevalence of Alzheimer's disease in a community population of older persons: Higher than previously reported. *Journal of the American Medical Association, 262,* 2551–2556.

Farran, C. J., & Keane-Hagerty, M. A. (1988). A group intervention program for caregivers of persons with dementia. In K. C. Buckwalter (Ed.), *Intervention strategies for maintaining control throughout the caregiving trajectory.* Iowa City, IA: Iowa Geriatric Education Center Interdisciplinary Monograph Series.

Fawcett, J. (1984). *Analysis and evaluation of conceptual models of nursing.* Philadelphia: F. A. Davis.

Feil, N. (1982). *Validation: The Feil method* (p.16). Cleveland, OH: Edward Feil Productions.

Foreman, M. (1986). Acute confusional states in hospitalized elderly: A research dilemma. *Nursing Research, 35,* 34–38.

Francis, G., & Baly, A. (1986). Plush animals: Do they make a difference? *Geriatric Nursing, 7,* 140–142.

Fruehwirth, S. S. (1989). An application of Johnson's behavioral model: A case study. *Journal of Community Health Nursing, 6,* 61–71.

Fryer, D. G. (1983). Summer dementia in the elderly. *Bulletin for the Mason Clinic, 37,* 67.

Gillies, D. A. (1986). Patients suffering from memory loss can be taught self-care. *Geriatric Nursing, 7,* 254–256.

Gillis, G., Whall, A., Booth, D., & Beel-Bates, C. (1989). *Disruptive behavior in elderly nursing home residents: A survey of nursing staff.* Presented at the 42nd Annual Gerontological Society of American Scientific Meeting. Minneapolis, MN.

Given, B. A., King, S. K., Collins, C., & Given, C. W. (1988). Family caregivers of the elderly: Involvement and reactions to care. *Archives of Psychiatric Nursing, II,* 281–288.

Gmeiner, C. (1987). Patient behavior, care needs, personalized community resources of both institutionalized and non-institutionalized Alzheimer's patients. In H. J. Altman (Ed.) *Alzheimer's disease: Problems, prospects, and perspectives,* (Proceedings of a National Conference on AD and Dementia, April, 1986). New York: Plenum Press.

Gomez, G., & Gomez, E. A. (1989). Dementia? Or Delirium? *Geriatric Nursing, 10,* 141–142.

Granow, J. L. (1988). *An in-home intervention program for caregivers of persons with dementia.* Iowa City, IA: Iowa Geriatric Education Center Interdisciplinary Monograph Series, 20–32.

Greene, J. A., Asp, J., & Crane, N. (1985). Specialized management of the Alzheimer's disease patient: Does it make a difference? *Journal of the Tennessee Medical Association.* Sept., 559–563.

Gueldner, S. H., & Hanner, M. B. (1989). Methodological issues related to gerontological nursing research. *Nursing Research, 38,* 183–185.

Hall, G. (1991). Altered thought processes: SDAT. In M. Maas & K. Buckwalter, (Eds.), *Nursing diagnoses and interventions for the elderly.* Menlo Park, CA: Addison Wesley.

Hall, G., & Buckwalter, K. (1987). Progressively lowered stress threshold: A conceptual model for care of adults with Alzheimer's Disease. *Archives of Psychiatric Nursing, 1,* 309–406.

Hall, G., Kirschling, V., & Todd, S. (1986). Sheltered freedom-an Alzheimer's unit in an ICF. *Geriatric Nursing, 7,* 132–137.

Haycox, J. A. (1984). A simple, reliable clinical behavioral scale for assessing demented patients. *Journal of Clinical Psychiatry, 45,* 23–24.

Hernandez, M., & Miller, J. (1986). How to reduce falls. *Geriatric Nursing, 7,* 97–102.

Heston, L., & White, J. (1983). *Dementia: A practical guide to Alzheimer's Disease and related illnesses.* New York: Freeman & Co.

Hing, E. (1987). Use of nursing homes by the elderly: Preliminary data from the 1985 National Nursing Home Survey. *National Gerontological Nursing Association Newsletter,* June/July.

Hogstel, M. D. (1979). Use of reality orientation with aging confused patients. *Nursing Research, 28,* 161–165.

Johnson, M., & Maguire, M. (1989). Give me a break: Benefits of a caregiver support service. *Journal of Gerontological Nursing, 15*(11), 22–26.

Jolles, J., & Hijman, R. (1983). The neuropsychology of aging and dementia. In W. H. Gispen & J. Traber (Eds.) *Aging of the brain. Developments in Neurology,* volume 7. New York: Elsevier Science.

Joske, W. D. (1974). Philosophy and the meaning of life. *Australian Journal of Philosophy, 52*(2), 93–104.

Kahana, E. (1975). A congruence model of person–environment interaction. In P. Windley, T. Byerts, & F. Ernst (Eds.), *Theory development in environment and aging.* Washington DC: Gerontological Society.

Kane, R. A., & Kane, R. L. (1981). *Assessing the elderly.* Lexington, MA: Lexington Books.

Katzman, R. (1986). Alzheimer's disease. *New England Journal of Medicine, 314,* 964–973.

King, I. M. (1971). *Toward a theory for nursing: General concepts of human behavior.* New York: Wiley.

Kongable, L., Buckwalter, K., & Stolley, J. (1989). The effects of pet therapy on the social behavior of institutionalized Alzheimer's clients. *Archives of Psychiatric Nursing, 3,* 191–198.

Kongable, L. G., Stolley, J. M., & Buckwalter, K. C. (1990). Pet therapy for Alzheimer's patients: A survey. *Journal of Long Term Care Administration, 18*(3), 17–21.

Kumar, V., Peterson, K., Kumar, N., & Fulk, L. (1989). Measuring cognitive and behavior changes in community dwelling Alzheimer's disease patients. *The American Journal of Alzheimer's Care and Related Disorders & Research, 4*(1), 13–18.

Langland, M., & Panicucci, C. (1982). Effects of touch on communication with elderly confused clients. *Journal of Gerontological Nursing, 8*(3), 152–155.

Lawton, M. P. (1975a). Competence, environmental press and the adaptation of older people. In P. Windley, T. Byerts, & F. Ernst (Eds.), *Theory development in environment and aging.* Washington DC: Gerontological Society.

Lawton, M. P. (1975b). The Philadelphia Geriatric Center Morale Scale: A revision. *Journal of Gerontology, 15,* 85–89.

Lawton, M. P. (1980). The lifespan of housing environments for the aging. *The Gerontologist, 20,* 56–64.

Libow, L. (1981). A rapidly administered, easily remembered mental status evaluation: FROMAJE., In L. S. Libow & F. T. Sherman, (Eds.), *The core of geriatric medicine.* St. Louis: Mosby.

Lincoln, R. (1984). What do nurses know about confusion in the aged? *Journal of Gerontological Nursing, 10*(8), 26–29.

Maas, M. (1988). Management of patients with Alzheimer's disease in long term care facilities. *Nursing Clinics of North America, 23*(1), 57–68.

Maas M., & Buckwalter, K. (1990). Final report, Nursing Evaluation Research: A Special Alzheimer's Unit National Institute of Health, National Center for Nursing Research. (#NR0689).

Maas, M., Buckwalter, K., & Kelley, L. (in press). Characteristics and perceptions of family members of institutionalized Alzheimer's patients. *Applied Nursing Research*.

Maas, M., & Hardy, M. (1988). Nursing diagnoses: A challenge for the future. *Journal of Gerontological Nursing, 14*(3), 8–13.

Mace, N., & Rabins, P. (1981). *The 36 hour day*. Baltimore, MD: Johns Hopkins University Press.

Mackey, M. (1983). OBS and nursing care. *Journal of Gerontological Nursing, 9*(2), 74–79, 83–85.

Matthew, L., Sloan, P., Kilby, M., & Flood, R. (1988). What's different about a special care unit for dementia patients? A comparative study. *Journal of Alzheimer's Care and Related Disorders and Research, 21*(2), 16–23.

Maxwell, R., Bader, J., & Watson, W. (1972). Territory and self in geriatric settings. *The Gerontologist, 12*, 413–417.

Mayers, K., & Griffin, M. (1990). The play project: Use of stimulus objects with demented patients. *Journal of Gerontological Nursing, 16*(1), 32–37.

McCracken A., & Fitzwater, E. (1989). The right environment for Alzheimer's. *Geriatric Nursing, 10*, 293–294.

McKhann, G., Drachman, D., Folstein, M., Katzman, R., Price, D., & Stadlan, E. (1984). Clinical diagnosis of Alzheimer's disease: Report of the NINCDS-ADRDA Work Group under the auspices of Department of Health and Human Services Task Force on Alzheimer's Disease. *Neurology, 34*, 939–944.

Meddaugh, D. (1991). Before aggression erupts. *Geriatric Nursing, 12*, 114–116.

Miller, D. B., Gulle N., & McCue, F. (1986). The realities of respite for families, clients, and sponsors. *The Gerontologist, 26*, 467–470.

Monsour, N., & Robb, S. (1982). Wandering behavior in old age: A psychosocial study. *Social Work, 27*, 411–416.

Moseley, P. W., Davies, H. D., & Priddy, J. M. (1988). Support groups for male caregivers of Alzheimer's patients: A followup. *Clinical Gerontologist, 7*, 127–136.

Neuman, B. W. (1982). *The Neuman Systems Model*. New York: Appleton-Century-Crofts.

Norberg, A., Melvin, E., & Asplund, K. (1986). Reactions to music, touch, and object presentation in the final stage of dementia: An exploratory study. *International Journal of Nursing Studies, 23*, 315–323.

Norberg, A., & Asplund, K. (1990). Caregivers' experience of caring for severely demented patients. *Western Journal of Nursing Research, 12*, 75–84.

Norberg, A., Asplund, K., & Waxman, H. (1987). Withdrawing feeding and withholding artificial nutrition from severely demented patients: Interviews with caregivers. *Western Journal of Nursing Research, 9*, 348–356.

Norberg, A., & Hirschfeld, M. (1987). Feeding of severely demented patients in institutions: Interviews with caregivers in Israel. *Journal of Advanced Nursing, 12*, 551–557.

O'Donnell, P., & Beck, C. (1987). *Biofeedback therapy of urinary incontinence in the elderly*. Presentation at the Sigma Theta Tau International Research Congress. Edinburgh, Scotland.

Office of Technological Assessment. (1987). Losing a Million Minds: Confronting the Tragedy of Alzheimer's Disease and Other Dementias. U.S. House of Representatives. Washington, DC: U.S. Government Printing Office.

Ohta, R., & Ohta, B. (1988). Special units for Alzheimer's disease patients: A critical look. *The Gerontologist, 28,* 803–808.

Orem, D. (1980). *Nursing: Concepts of practice.* New York: McGraw-Hill.

Orlando, I. J. (1961). *The dynamic nurse-patient relationship.* New York: G. P. Putnam's Sons.

Pajik, M. (1984). Alzheimer's disease: Inpatient care. *American Journal of Nursing, 2,* 215–222, 232.

Palmateer, L. M., & McCartney, J. R. (1985). Do nurses know when patients have cognitive deficits? *Journal of Gerontological Nursing, 11*(2), 6–16.

Peplau, H. E. (1952). *Interpersonal relations in nursing.* New York: G. P. Putnam's Sons.

Peterson, R. F., Knapp, R., Rosen, J. C., & Pither, B. F. (1977). The effects of furniture arrangements on the behavior of geriatric patients. *Behavior Therapy, 8,* 464–467.

Phillips, L. R., & Rempusheski, V. F. (1986). Caring for the frail elderly at home: Toward a theoretical explanation of the dynamics of poor family caregiving. *Advances in Nursing Science, 8*(4), 62–84.

Phillips, L. R., Rempusheski, V. F., & Morrison, E. (1989). Developing and testing beliefs about caregiving scale. *Research in Nursing and Health, 12,* 207–220.

Plutchik, R., Conte, H., Lieberman, M., Bakur, M., Grossman, J., & Lehrman, N. (1970). Reliability and validity of a scale for assessing the functioning of geriatric patients. *Journal of the American Geriatrics Society, 18,* 491–500.

Pratt, C., Schmall, V., Wright, S., & Hare, D. (1987). Ethical concerns of family caregivers to dementia patients. *The Gerontologist, 27,* 632–638.

Quayhagen, M. P., & Quayhagen, M. (1988). Alzheimer's stress: Coping with the caregiving role. *The Gerontologist, 28,* 391–396.

Quayhagen, M. P., & Quayhagen, M., (1989). Differential effects of family-based strategies on Alzheimer's Disease. *The Gerontologist, 29,* 150–155.

Rabins, P. V., Mace, M. A., & Lucas, M. J. (1982). The impact of dementia on the family. *Journal of the American Medical Association, 248,* 333–335.

Rameizl, P. (1983). CADET: A self assessment tool. *Journal of Gerontological Nursing, 4,* 377–378.

Rheaume, Y., Riley, M. S., & Volicer, L. (1987). Meeting nutritional needs of Alzheimer's patients who pace constantly. *Journal of Nutrition for the Elderly, 7,* 43–52.

Ricci, M. (1983). All-out care for an Alzheimer's patient. *Geriatric Nursing, 4,* 369–371.

Ridder, M. (1985). Nursing update on Alzheimer's disease. *Journal of Neurosurgical Nursing. 17,* 190–200.

Robb, S., Stegman, C., & Wolanin, M. (1986). No research versus research with compromised results: A study of validation therapy. *Nursing Research, 35,* 113–118.

Roberts, B. L., & Algase, D. L. (1988). Victims of Alzheimer's disease and the environment. *Nursing Clinics of North America, 35*(2), 113–118.

Rogers, M. E. (1970). *The theoretical basis of nursing.* Philadelphia: Davis.

Rosswurm, M. A. (1989). Assessment of perceptual processing deficits in persons with Alzheimer's disease. *Western Journal of Nursing Research, 11,* 458–468.

Rosswurm, M. A., Zimmerman, S., Schwartz-Fulton, J., & Norman, G. (1986). Can we manage wandering behavior? *The Journal of Long-Term Care Administration, 14*(3), 5–8.

Roy, C. (1984). *Introduction to nursing: An adaptation model.* Englewood Cliffs, NJ: Prentice-Hall.

Roy, C., & Roberts, S. (1981). *Theory construction in nursing: An adaptation model.* Englewood Cliffs, NJ: Prentice-Hall.

Ryden, M. B. (1988). Aggressive behavior in persons with dementia who live in the community. *Alzheimer's Disease and Associated Disorders, 2,* 342–355.

Sandman, P. O., Norberg, A., Adolfsson, R., Axelsson, K., & Hedly, V. (1986). Morning care of patients with Alzheimer-type dementia. A theoretical model based on direct observations. *Journal of Advanced Nursing, 11,* 369–378.

Schmidt, G. L., & Keyes, B. (1985). Group psychotherapy with family caregivers of demented patients. *The Gerontologist, 25,* 347–349.

Schwab, M., Rader, J., & Doan, J. (1985). Relieving the anxiety and fear in dementia. *Journal of Gerontological Nursing, 11*(5), 8–15.

Shoemaker, D. (1987). Problematic behavior and the Alzheimer's patient: Retrospection as a method of understanding and counseling. *The Gerontologist, 27,* 370–374.

Silverstone, B., & Burach-Weiss, A. (1983). *Social work practice with the frail elderly and their families: The Auxilliary Function Model.* Springfield, IL: Thomas.

Snyder, L. H., Rupprecht, P. A., Pyret, J., Brekhus, S., & Moss, T. (1978). Wandering. *The Gerontologist, 18,* 272–280.

Steffes, R., & Thralow, J. (1985). Do uniform colors keep patients awake? *Journal of Gerontological Nursing, 11*(7), 6–9.

Stommel, M., Given, C., & Given, B. (1990). Depression as an overriding variable explaining caregiver burdens. *Journal of Aging and Health, 2,* 81–102.

Warren, J. W., Sobal, J., Tenney, J. H., Hoppes, J. M., Damron, D., Levenson, S., DeForge, B. R., & Muncie, H. L. (1986). Informed consent by proxy: An issue in research with elderly patients. *New England Journal of Medicine, 315,* 1124–1128.

Wilson, H. S. (1989). Family caregivers: The experience of Alzheimer's disease. *Applied Nursing Research, 2,* 40–45.

Wolanin, M., & Phillips, L. (1981). *Confusion: Prevention and care.* St. Louis: Mosby.

Woods, R. (1982). The psychiatry of aging: Assessment of defects and their management. In R. Levy & F. Post (Eds.), *The psychology of latter life* (pp. 68–113). Boston: Blackwell Scientific.

Young, S. H., Muir-Nash, J., & Ninos, M. (1988). Managing nocturnal wandering behavior. *Journal of Gerontological Nursing, 14*(5), 6–12.

Zarit, S. H. (1989a). Do we need another "stress and caregiving" study? *The Gerontologist, 29,* 147–148.

Zarit, S. H. (1989b). Issues and directions in family intervention research. In E. Light & B. D. Lebowitz (Eds.), *Alzheimer's Disease Treatment and Family Stress: Directions for Research.* Rockville, MD: National Institute of Mental Health, U.S. Department of Health and Human Services.

Chapter 3

Human Responses to Catastrophe

SHIRLEY A. MURPHY
SCHOOL OF NURSING
UNIVERSITY OF WASHINGTON
SEATTLE, WASHINGTON

CONTENTS

Human responses to catastrophic events are defined as social and mental constructions of reality in which a relatively self-sufficient part of a community undergoes severe loss or threat of loss to its members (Wilkinson, 1985). In this chapter, catastrophic illness research includes epidemics of rapid transmission such as infectious and food-borne diseases. Research on cata-

57

strophic events includes study of the effects of natural and technological disasters on various populations. Threat-of-catastrophe or "invisible trauma" research includes threat of nuclear war and accidents, threat of leakage of toxic chemical spills, and unknown health effects of pesticides.

As a direct result of a catastrophe, social structure is disrupted to the extent that ongoing essential functions are prevented or delayed. Affected are survival (health, shelter, emotional equilibrium); social order (provision of vital services, cultural norms, proscribed and prescribed role functioning); and systems of meaning (values, shared definitions of reality, communication). The goals of this integrative review are to summarize and critically review accumulated knowledge and to highlight important issues unresolved to date. This review is limited by the lack of nursing research focused on catastrophic loss. Therefore, it was impossible to report studies in an integrative format in some sections.

PROCESS OF REVIEW

Thirteen journals were examined for review from 1980 through 1988: *Advances in Nursing Science, Archives of Psychiatric Nursing, Image: The Journal of Nursing Scholarship, Journal of Scholarly Inquiry, International Journal of Mass Emergencies and Disasters, International Journal of Nursing Research, Issues in Mental Health Nursing, Journal of Advanced Nursing, Journal of Professional Nursing, Journal of Traumatic Stress, Nursing Research, Public Health Nursing, Research in Nursing & Health,* and *Western Journal of Nursing Research.* Additional research reports were found in selected journals and books in which articles on the topics of interest were known to the author.

Inclusion criteria were: (a) the purpose of the article had to be a systematic inquiry that included a problem statement, background/rationale, a description of methods, results, and conclusion; and (b) if the article was written by a single author, it had to be a nurse; multiple-authored reports had to include a nurse author. Some articles may have been missed if nurse authors were not designated by credentials, title, or affiliation.

CONCEPTUAL FRAMEWORK

A model of human responses to catastrophes is used to organize the literature. The model, selected to illustrate human responses to catastrophes at individual, organizational, or community levels, delineates seven sets of empirically based factors shown to be important in the study of catastrophic phenomena: preexisting factors, event factors, stress-appraisal factors, mediating factors, immediate responses, short-term effects, and long-term outcomes. The "community" level of analysis is the most difficult to describe. For example, an airplane crash has implications for the local "community" of rescue workers and nonpassengers. Depending on how an incident unfolds, the victims may become a "community." Airplane disaster victims also have a social network elsewhere. No attempt is made to link events or catastrophic illness to national or international communities in this review.

Preexisting Factors

Constructs and their empirical indicators in this dimension can be operationalized at the individual, organizational, or community level, depending on the study undertaken. For example, constructs at the individual level could include demographic and individual trait factors shown to influence stress appraisal, coping, and adaptation (Boatright, 1985; Bugen, 1977; Hyman & Woog, 1982; Lazarus & Folkman, 1984; Logue, Melick, & Struening, 1981). Organizational constructs could be leadership, job demand, or job decision latitude (Karasek, 1979; Matteson & Ivancevich, 1987). Community constructs could be level of community preparedness for outbreak of contagion or disaster and past experience with traumatic events (Hardin & Cohen, 1988; Meisenhelder & LaCharite, 1989).

Event Factors

Constructs that might be studied here include the nature of transmission of illness, the scope and duration of impact of an illness or loss event, and the type of causal agent, that is, natural or technological disasters. In the case of threatened catastrophe, accuracy, availability, and timing of release of information about a phenomenon would be important. Event factors are not stressors per se, rather it is one's perception of events that define them as stressors (Kreps, 1978; Pilisuk & Acredolo, 1988).

Stress Appraisal Factors

At the individual level, primary, secondary, and reappraisal processes conceptualized by Lazarus and Folkman (1984) are useful. It is the individual's appraisal process that determines whether an event is benign or stressful, that is, meaning is constructed by evaluating whether the stressor is viewed as harmful, a loss, a threat, or a challenge. At the organizational and community levels, assessment of disruption of services, economic costs, and ability to institute emergency plans might be defined and studied.

Mediating Factors

At the individual level, factors known to mediate the effects of stress on health status are one's system of coping and resources available, both interpersonal and material (Murphy, 1987; Norbeck, 1988). At the organizational level, debriefing of critical incidents is a strategy that has potential for study (Mitchell, 1983). At the community level, readiness to respond is an important factor (Glittenberg, 1981).

Outcomes

Because of the nature of catastrophic phenomena, immediate, short-, and long-term responses should be considered. Responses can be conceptualized for all three levels of analysis. For example, at the individual level, short-term responses could include physiological, cognitive, and behavioral constructs (Cohen et al., 1988). Immediate responses at the organizational level might be a hospital's system for contacting employees for crisis intervention (Miles, Demi, & Mostyn-Aker, 1984). At the community level, long-term responses frequently studied include the impact of rumors and false information on recovery and economic impact (Wenger, 1978).

CATASTROPHIC ILLNESS: 1980 to 1988

Preventive health actions including immunizations, education, and legislation of hygenic practices have limited infectious diseases. However, recent media reports suggested that relaxation of preventive actions may increase incidence and hence the need to investigate infectious diseases. According to television reports, 25% to 40% of all U.S. children under the age of four are currently not immunized. Moreover, outbreaks of measles on university campuses in 1988 and 1989 attest to increased incidence of preventable, but rapidly transmittable communicable diseases.

In 1981 epidemiologists cautioned that Human Immunodeficiency Virus (HIV), and its extreme form, Acquired Immunodeficiency Syndrome (AIDS) may reach epidemic proportions. By 1987, there were about 43,000 cases diagnosed in the United States (Center for Disease Control [CDC], 1987).

Variations of the proposed conceptual model are appropriate to guide studies of catastrophic illness. Of the catastrophic illness studies reviewed, only one included a theoretical framework.

Prototypical Illnesses

Human Responses to Food-Borne Botulism.   Cohen et al. (1988) used a crisis model to develop a longitudinal study of immediate and long-term effects of food-borne botulism on both victims and their families. The investigators reported the event to be the third largest outbreak of this illness in the United States. All of the study participants (28 victims and 51 family members) perceived the experience as an acute situational crisis. The effects were both life-threatening and psychosocially devastating. In the first patient study reported, the major variable of interest, daily functioning, was measured by the Sickness Impact Profile (SIP) (Gilson et al., 1975) at 4, 8, 12, 18, 24, and 36 months posthospitalization. The mean length of hospital stay was 50 days; 12 patients were on ventilators for an average of 68 days. The investigators found that regardless of physical impairment, all patients reported long-lasting psychosocial effects, particularly depression.

In a second publication reporting findings of food-borne botulism, Hardin and Cohen (1988) described psychosocial effects over time on both victims and their families. During lengthy stays in critical care areas, patients reported feelings of depersonalization and perceptions that discussion of their feelings was not welcomed by either family members or nurses. Death anxiety was reported by 82% of the sample, and depression was reported by 91% up to the third anniversary of the event. Anger over severe physical disability was also widespread.

Fifty-one first degree relatives (immediate family members) participated in the family component of the study. Variables of interest were family functioning, including role substitution for the ill family members, perceived emotional support provided to victims, and mental health status, specifically anxiety and depression. Data were collected by audiotaped interviews in family homes approximately 1 and 2 years after the outbreak and by videotaped group meetings that included patients, families, nursing staff, and the research team 3 years after the event. The investigators found that family members experienced anxiety regarding home care responsibilities and expressed "terror at seeing someone change from perfect health to being paralyzed." Unlike victims, family members tended to avoid disclosure of feelings and did not report high levels of depression. Adaptation required negotiation and restructuring of family role commitments.

The strengths of the Cohen et al. (1988) and Hardin and Cohen (1988) studies included the inclusion of a theoretical framework, a thorough review of the literature, the longitudinal design, unique data-collection methods, and rapid dissemination of findings. Limitations difficult to overcome included the small sample and the lack of a comparison group for the family component of the study. An additional weakness of the study was the use of a crisis model in a study that examined coping, adaptation, and health outcomes over a three-year period. The scope of the study was not impeded by the framework; rather the framework was too restrictive to embrace all of the important study parameters.

Human Responses to HIV-Related Illnesses. Williams, D'Aquila, and Williams (1987) surveyed 181 heterosexual intravenous drug users, who had entered treatment to determine seroprevalence of HIV infection in this high-risk group. Study variables of interest were drug abuse history, treatment history, sexual behaviors, and demographic characteristics. At the time of the survey, 65% had already decreased needle-sharing behavior and 98% were using needle-cleaning techniques. Risk factors that differentiated seropositive from seronegative persons were ethnicity (Black or Hispanic), age (over 30), and history (over 10 years of drug use).

Lovejoy and Moran (1988) obtained data from a convenience sample of 30 homosexual or bisexual men who had symptomatic progression of AIDS and met specific criteria. The AIDS Beliefs and Behaviors Questionnaire (McKusick, 1985) modified by the authors was used to collect data. Results indicated that 90% wanted more information about the immune system, whereas only 10% wanted explicit information about safe sexual behavior.

A third descriptive study reported by Barrick (1988) assessed the willingness of nursing personnel to care for AIDS patients. Study participants were employed in a single urban hospital in a Western state and were surveyed by mail. Anonymous questionnaires were returned by 208 (44%) bedside nursing personnel. The majority of responders (88%) were female registered nurses averaging 12 years experience. Data were collected by a 13-item, investigator-developed instrument that assessed willingness to care for AIDS patients and a standardized instrument, Attitudes Toward Lesbians and Gay Men (Herick, 1985). The researchers found (a) a statistically significant correlation between attitudes toward lesbians and gay men and willingness to care for AIDS patients ($r = .50, p < .01$); (b) a 25% covariance between negative attitudes and unwillingness to care for AIDS patients ($r^2 = .25$, p value not reported); (c) women participants were significantly more anti-homosexual than men (t value not reported, p < .01); (d) 25% of the respondents felt that AIDS patients should be quarantined, and (e) 9% said they would refuse assignment to a patient with AIDS.

The studies on AIDS demonstrated a beginning attempt by nurse investigators to study the complex problems associated with AIDS and related syndromes. Major limitations of all three studies were the absence of a theoretical rationale for the research and the lack of standardized measurement tools. Replication and extension of these studies should incorporate comparison groups, larger samples, and control of threats to internal and external validity.

CATASTROPHIC EVENTS: 1980 TO 1988

In recent years, investigators in several behavioral science and health disciplines have become interested in studying long-term health and adaptive consequences of many types of disasters. Studies of the Buffalo Creek disaster in Pennsylvania in the late 1970s mark the beginning of carefully controlled studies that assessed multiple outcomes of recovery. The hallmark of these studies and of several since is that some victims have demonstrated negative health and adaptive consequences and have been compensated for their losses.

Disasters are massive stress situations and generally are conceptualized by their causative agents, natural (viewed as acts of God) and technological; both are reported in this review. This classification of disasters is not mutually exclusive. Although airplane crashes and community acts of violence can also be termed disasters, no current classification scheme includes these events. Threat of catastrophe, or situations of overwhelming threat to well-being, need to be tested with adjustments to classic stress/coping/adaptation models. In order to examine selected studies, several definitions may be useful.

The Disaster Relief Act of 1974 defined major natural disaster. Included were "any hurricane, tornado, storm, flood, high-water, wind-driven water, tidal wave, tsunami, earthquake, volcanic eruption, landslide, snow storm, drought, fire, explosion, or other catastrophe in any part of the continental United States, or its territories, which causes damage of sufficient severity and magnitude to warrant major disaster assistance" (U.S. Public Health Service, 1976).

There is no official consensual definition of technological disasters. However, they have some salient characteristics that may or may not differentiate them from natural disasters. Examples are hotel fires, airplane crashes, nuclear reactor accidents, and the dumping of toxic wastes. Subjective appraisal is an important consideration in technological or "man-made" events. For example, the extent to which one believes an incident could have been prevented may have a direct relationship to the amount of anger and blame generated. The extent to which hostile feelings are expressed may affect mental health outcomes. It may be that if blame can be attributed to a specific person or organization, more energy is devoted to seeking retribution rather than to integrating the event into the life experience. Errors in human judgment that ultimately harm others evoke responses contrary to human values. Alternatively, if one believes events such as hurricanes and tornadoes are caused by an agent over which one has no control (i.e., atmospheric processes), it may be that victims will formulate the attribution, "nothing could be done." Recovery is reportedly less stressful following natural disasters; however, the human factors associated with adequate warning and rescue operations are indeed present, and hence, may be sources of error that also result in beliefs that the consequences could have been less damaging. Thus, both natural and technological events involve potential human error, which points up an important similarity between the two kinds of disasters. At the present time, little comparative analysis of events caused by different causative agents has been done.

There is a general lack of agreement among researchers regarding estimates of physical and mental health consequences following disaster. According to Melick (1985): (a) mental health consequences are more likely than physical health consequences, (b) controlled studies that assess mental health consequences using standardized instruments report lower rates of impairment than studies that obtain data by interview and collect no comparative data, (c) rescue workers exhibit similar consequences and should also be viewed as disaster victims, and (d) the majority of victims are reluctant to take advantage of mental health services. Twelve research papers are reviewed in this section. The studies are grouped into five major categories: (a) victim health status and recovery, (b) rescue worker response, (c) indirect effects on significant others, (d) community response/reorganization, and (e) methodological studies.

Victim Health Status and Recovery

Four studies involved adults; one involved children. Stress and coping models provided the theoretical basis for all five studies. Conceptual linkages among selected variables were hypothesized and tested. Detailed examples of these models can be found in several published papers (Hartsough, 1985; Logue, Melick & Struening, 1981; Murphy, 1989a).

Description of Events.   Melick (1976) and Logue (1978) studied health consequences longitudinally following Tropical Storm Agnes that occurred in 1972. An estimated 116,000 homes were destroyed, public property damage was estimated at $700 million, and 118 persons died. Melick's study (1976) was conducted 3 years postdisaster. The sample included 43 flood and 48 nonflood working class men. In a related study, Logue (1978) studied 407 flood and 155 nonflood female respondents 5 years postdisaster. Both studies were designed to examine life changes at several points in time, before and after the flood.

Murphy (1984, 1986a, 1986b, 1987) studied stress, coping, and health outcomes 1 and 3 years following the 1981 volcanic eruption of Mount St. Helens in southwestern Washington state. Sixty persons were known or presumed dead and both private and public property damage was extensive. A unique feature of the disaster was that death and property loss were mutually exclusive except in a few cases, which allowed the investigator to study two types of bereavement, two types of property loss, and a nondisaster loss comparison group ($n = 155$). Several secondary analysis studies evolved from the data set. Cowan and Murphy (1985) focused on 69 bereaved respondents.

Boatright (1985) conducted a longitudinal study of psychological effects on children following the 1974 Xenia, Ohio tornado. Psychological effects were conceptualized as school absenteeism among second to sixth graders ($n = 47$) whose school was destroyed. The comparison group consisted of children ($n = 75$) enrolled in the same grades in a school 14 miles away and not affected by the tornado.

Subjective Appraisals of Events. In the four studies in which researchers collected data from adults, subjective reactions also were assessed. Examples of subjective appraisal in these studies included the impact of the loss of a family member, damage to one's home, moving into temporary housing, unemployment, economic loss, disruption in social networks, and lifestyle change. Appraisals were made by standarized measures such as The Schedule of Recent Experiences (Hawkins, Davies, & Holmes, 1957) and the Life Experiences Survey (Sarason, Johnson, & Siegel, 1978).

Mediating Variables. Factors suggested to mediate the relationship between stressful life events and health and recovery at the individual level of analysis have been proposed by Hyman and Woog (1982), Lazarus and Folkman (1984), and others. Three major categories have been suggested: personal, social, and economic resources. In the studies reported here, investigators conceptualized personal resources as coping strategies (Logue et al., 1981; Murphy, 1986b) and self-efficacy (Murphy, 1987). Social resources were conceptualized as social network size and structure, religious and community support, and perceptions of available support. Economic resources were conceptualized as employment status, government aid, and changes in income. These data were collected by standardized measures and by items developed by investigators.

Measures of Health Outcome and Recovery. Multiple approaches measuring the same construct are recommended for enhancing precision and increasing theory development in psychological/emotional effects of disaster (Hartsough, 1985; Green, 1982). Both mental and physical health outcomes and perceptions of recovery were measured by multiple standardized instruments and investigator-developed items in the adult studies (Logue et al., 1981; Murphy, 1984; 1986a; 1986b; 1987). Boatright (1985) obtained school attendance records to document absenteeism as a measure of psychological effects of disaster on children in her sample.

Comparability of Findings. It is possible to make comparisons across the adult studies because the mental and physical health dependent variables were measured by the same instruments: the Symptom Checklist 90 (SCL-90) (Derogatis, 1977) and a 50-item symptom checklist obtained by the National Center for Health Statistics, United States Department of Health, Education, & Welfare (USDHEW, 1975).

In the adult studies, all disaster loss groups reported higher rates of emotional distress than comparison groups; however, scores did not reach statistical significance in the Melick (1976) and Logue (1978) studies. In the Murphy (1986b) and Cowan and Murphy (1985) studies, scores were statistically significant for all loss groups one year postdisaster and for the combined (presumed and confirmed dead) bereaved group three years postdisaster. Differences in the findings between the three studies referred to in this paragraph may be attributed to timing of data collection and within sample comparisons made in the Murphy (1986b) study.

Physical health findings were opposite those of mental health findings. Statistically significant differences were noted between loss and nonloss groups in the Melick (1976) and Logue (1978) studies, but not in the Murphy (1986b) and Cowan and Murphy (1985) studies.

In the Boatright (1985) study findings regarding absenteeism rates among second to sixth graders in disaster and nondisaster school districts, the investigation found no significant differences 1½ months postdisaster, but significant differences 8 and 14 months postdisaster. There were no significant differences by gender. Several limitations were pointed out by the investigator: (a) absenteeism for other causes was not controlled, (b) the experimental group had to change schools and travel additional miles, (c) absenteeism is only one indicator of psychological distress in children, and (d) the sample was small.

Secondary Effects on Families

A second more recent line of catastrophic event research pertains to the identification of posttraumatic stress disorder (PTSD) as a dependent variable. PTSD is defined by the American Psychiatric Association (1980) as: (a) the experience of a stressor severe enough to cause significant symptoms of reexperience and avoidance in almost anyone; (b) reexperience of the stressor in at least one of three modes, that is, dreams, intrusive thoughts; (c) avoidance phenomena in at least one of three modes, that is, feeling detached from others; and (d) at least two of six related symptoms, for example, guilt, sleep disturbance. The Vietnam veteran population has been studied extensively. However studies on the effects of the Vietnam experience on the family of those in military service in Vietnam are recent extensions of stress/coping/PTSD models. One study that met review criteria was found.

Verbosky and Ryan (1988) studied female partners of Vietnam veterans.

A convenience sample consisted of 23 women partners of Vietnam veterans who were attending significant others therapy groups. The groups were 8 to 12 weeks long, time-limited and close-ended. The women were young (age range 24 to 38 years). Most had been married 2 to 19 years; the remainder had cohabitated with veterans 1 to 7 years. All were employed full-time, with half the sample holding two jobs. The women sought therapy for four major partner-related stressors: (a) inability to tolerate substance abuse, (b) physical abuse, (c) difficulty coping with PTSD symptoms, and (d) ambivalence around remaining in the relationship. Data were collected by reviewing group process notes around these four stressors. The investigators found that trying to manage PTSD symptoms in partners was the most frequently identified stressor. Partners' isolation, rage, and inability to contribute to daily living responsibilities were consistent themes. PTSD symptoms in the study sample consisted of guilt, lack of emotional involvement, and inability to control or change partner behaviors, such as nightmares. There are numerous limitations of the study, such as potential bias in sampling only those in treatment, the lack of a comparison group, and the lack of documentation of validity and reliability of data collection and analysis procedures. However, it represents a beginning attempt to study secondary effects of stressful experiences on family members.

Disaster Emergency Personnel

Disaster emergency personnel viewed as victims is a recent phenomenon receiving systematic study only in the past decade. The "worker as victim" experiences both similar and different stresses and outcomes when compared with other disaster victims. Regarding similarities, they are exposed to stressors that put them at risk for both mental and physical illness and they perceive no need for intervention. In terms of differences, emergency personnel experience occupational hazards such as high job demand and low job decision latitude—a combination, according to Karasek (1979), that produces high job-related stress. Second, the skills required to maintain competency have to be performed frequently enough for personnel to perceive competence, but infrequently enough to prevent burnout.

Because of the unique demands of emergency personnel, studies of their human responses should be based on conceptual models of occupational stress, such as that proposed by Matteson and Ivancevich (1987) or LaRocco, House, and French (1980). These models provide for conceptualization of both organizational and extra-organizational stressors and their outcomes so that empirical indicators can be identified and measured separately. Two studies of disaster personnel were found in which nurses were investigators. *Description of Events Studied.* Laube (1985) conducted a unique study of health care providers' responses to the 1974 Xenia, Ohio tornado. Thirty-four persons were killed; 78% of the community residents were treated at local hospitals, and over 3,000 homes and businesses were destroyed or severely damaged in the small community of 22,700 persons. The study goals were to: (a) determine the extent to which health care providers experienced role conflict in deciding whether to respond to the community crisis or to assist one's own family, and (b) determine the long-term health effects of workers regardless of role selected. Family/community conflict referred to the forced choice that must be made by individual family members who have well-defined and important disaster roles in the community, such as health care work. Data pertaining to role enactment were collected by interview within 11 days postdisaster. The sample consisted of 101 health care providers, (49 registered nurses and 52 physicians, laboratory technicians, and aides). The mean age of the sample, including a small comparison group ($n =$ 17), was 37 years.

In the second study, Miles, Demi, and Mostyn-Aker (1984) studied rescue workers' responses to a technological disaster, the 1981 Kansas City, Missouri, Hyatt-Regency Hotel skywalk collapse. This disaster left 114 persons dead and 188 injured. The investigators were interested in describing the emotional and physical sequalae of emergency personnel both on- and off-site. The study sample consisted of 54 rescue workers. Fifty percent were firemen and nurses; the remaining 50% were various health and nonhealth care workers. The average age of the sample was also 37 years.

Both studies measured emotional response outcomes using standardized instruments. Laube (1974, 1985) used the Psychiatric Status Schedule (PSS) (Spitzer, Endicott, Fleiss, & Cohen, 1970). She interviewed health care workers between 1 and 11 days postdisaster in order to obtain role conflict decision data. Miles et al. (1984) used the 58-item version of the Symptom Checklist (Derogatis, Lipman, Rickels, Uehlenhuth, & Covi, 1974). In addition, Miles et al. (1984) obtained measures of physical health, occupational role, and demographic data from investigator-developed measures 4 months postdisaster.

Findings.   In Laube's (1974, 1985) study, family and community role conflict data were analyzed by gender. Of the female subsample ($n = 81$), 50% had family responsibilities and chose family roles, that is, decided to remain with family during the event; 26% had family responsibilities but chose community roles, that is, went to employing hospital; and the remainder, who had no family responsibilities, chose community roles. For the male subsample ($n = 20$), 41% had family responsibilities and chose family roles, 47% had family responsibilities but chose community roles, and the remainder had no family responsibilities and all elected community roles. Participants were then grouped according to role conflict status and role participation for analysis of PSS scores. Emotional distress scores were higher for health care providers who had role conflict and chose community over family roles; however scores were in the normal range. Two years later, those who had role conflict reported significant increases in subjective stress regardless of role selected, whereas those who had no family responsibilities had reduced stress scores. Laube cautions that these findings must be interpreted with caution since less than 50% responded to the follow-up.

Miles et al. (1984) reported no significant differences in mental distress in their sample when scores were compared with normative sample scores. Nonetheless, 33% of the sample sought help from family, friends, and coworkers to cope with distress, and 28% sought professional counseling. Increases in physical health symptoms and in the use of alcohol, caffeine, tranquilizers, and tobacco also were reported. The investigators urged caution in interpretation of findings because subject selection was nonrandom, small, and no comparison group was included.

Community Responses

Community responses to disaster involve assessment of economic impact, interruption of expected services, provision of additional emergency services, and development of a sociopolitical climate for rebuilding and restoration. Community response studies are more typical than individual response studies and have been widely reported.

Community models of response to disaster have been developed by Wenger (1978), Dynes (1970), and Kreps (1978). In these models, communities are conceptualized as problem-solving entities. Linkages between community structure and contextual factors (e.g., disaster experience, crisis management capabilities), type of disaster, and disaster impact on recovery can be identified and measured.

Glittenberg (1981, 1985) was a member of an interdisciplinary team that conducted a longitudinal study following the 1976 earthquake in Guatemala. She used a stress framework to study the process of community recovery of four very poor urban settlements hit hardest by the disaster. The earthquake was responsible for 25,000 deaths, 75,000 serious injuries, and a million homeless. Each settlement was inhabited by 10,000 to 15,000 people who lost all their homes and possessions. The settlements studied were compared according to reconstruction plan: forced, planned, or unplanned. Reconstruction, the dependent variable, was defined as change in level of living over a 5-year period and was measured by four predictor variables: decision-making, leadership style, social matrix, and psychological status of respondents. The investigator found that the planned settlements that received the most aid earliest had the highest rates of recovery. However, by the end of the 5-year period, the unplanned and forced settlements were achieving similar states of recovery, but not without visible effects of low-level participation, helplessness, and anomie. Glittenberg concluded that all aid given was important, but that permanent, safe housing was the most significant.

Methodological Studies

Two published methodological studies were found. Both studies resulted from the Mt. St. Helens volcano data set. The first was undertaken to demonstrate that scores from pairs of bereaved study participants were independent; that is, not related, which is contrary to traditional measurement of paired data. The investigators found no statistically significant relationships between pairs of subjects on any major study variables (Murphy & Stewart, 1985–1986). Subsequently, Kiger (1984) conducted a longitudinal reliability study of the Symptom Checklist 90-R (SCL-90-R) using a contrasted groups approach to evaluate internal consistency and test stability of the instrument (Kiger & Murphy, 1987). Kiger found that for both the bereaved and comparison groups and at both 1 and 3 years postdisaster, coefficient alphas were 0.95. Tests for stability showed the same pattern of results. Coefficients ranged from $r = .47$ to $r = .69$, significant at $p < .001$.

THREAT OF CATASTROPHE: 1980 TO 1988

A final category of studies reviewed that belong to the general stress/coping/adaptation taxonomy are threat of catastrophe, sometimes referred to as invisible traumas or nonevents. Increasingly, these phenomena are responsible for extreme personal and community grief and loss. Threats of catastrophe include threats of nuclear war, threats of accidents at nuclear power plants, threats of leakage of toxic chemical and nuclear waste, and unknown effects of pesticides. The health and social consequences of these potentially life-threatening events may not appear until decades later. Soil contamination may poison the food supply, yet some persons never experience symptoms; those who do show widespread variation. According to Pilisuk and Acredolo (1988), the difference between individuals who have no visible effects and those who become ill may depend on the degree of exposure to other environmental risk factors such as smoking or living downwind from a chemical complex.

Of interest to nursing science is how individuals construct schemata to understand invisible danger, potential exposure, the ambiguity of the relationship between exposure and health consequences, and endure suffering that is devoid of meaning. Current conceptualizations of stress do not consider attributional theory, such as the roles of blame and responsibility. Additional constructs of interest are uncertainty, information-processing, and decision-making.

Threats of Contamination and Contagion

The one threat of catastrophe study that met inclusion criteria was that of Stanitis and Winder (1986). They used a health belief model to examine nurses' beliefs about nuclear war avoidance. The investigators surveyed 156 nurses employed in health care and educational institutions in the Northeast. The mean age of the sample was 44 years, 83% favored the 1982 American Nurses' Association (ANA) position on the prevention of nuclear war, and 28% were active in opposition to nuclear war. A 25-item questionnaire pertaining to U.S./Soviet relations, the use of nuclear weapons, and the future was adapted to fit the health belief model. Content validity was established by expert raters. Coefficient alpha was 0.85. Anonymous responses were obtained from 54% of those contacted. The researchers found that personal susceptibility, concern for benefits over costs, and attention to cues to action characterize nurses who believe in personal action. However, these beliefs were not predictive of potential action to prevent nuclear war. Moreover, professional organization membership, agreement with the ANA position, and parental status were not predictive of actions to avoid nuclear war.

FUTURE RESEARCH DIRECTIONS

The research reviewed in this chapter demonstrates creativity, yet limitations in both quantity and quality. Several reasons may account for the paucity of studies in this conceptual domain. First, access to study populations has been limited in part due to the unavailability of sufficient funding that can be obtained quickly. Some of the initial data collections of longitudinal studies reported in this review were doctoral dissertations (Laube, 1974; Logue, 1978; Melick, 1976; Murphy, 1982), which provided some monetary and material resources, such as consultation and computer access. Since the mid 1980s, the National Science Foundation and the National Institute of Mental Health have adopted "quick response" formats that allow entry into the field soon enough to obtain immediate response data that serves as a basis for additional research proposal development.

Second, catastrophic illnesses of the scope and impact of the past such as the Plague in the 14th Century have disappeared. In their place are illnesses resulting from changing mores, such as genital herpes and illnesses of rapid transmission such as botulism, communicable diseases, and AIDS. These illnesses and those that arise from pesticides, contamination, and chemical warfare agents are more recent phenomena that nurses have not yet studied extensively. Thus, current gaps in knowledge are widespread.

Gaps in knowledge are evident in all dimensions of the proposed conceptual model. Although many constructs have been identified and defined in all dimensions of the model, the data collected are primarily descriptive. Few linkages among constructs have been hypothesized and tested. Replication and extension studies are nonexistent.

Only one test of theory was found for this review. Laube's (1974, 1985) study of role conflict among care providers was a test of deductive theory.

A second deficit in tests of deductive theory pertains to adult development. None of the studies reviewed attempted to link catastrophic loss with developmental tasks of adulthood nor investigate the extent to which loss impedes, promotes, or does not affect adult development.

A third and somewhat surprising deficit is the lack of inductive theory development. Many nurse scholars are advocates of grounded theory and phenomenological approaches to scientific inquiry.

Some of the studies reviewed here are important first steps, but need to be followed up rapidly by quasi-experimental, longitudinal designs with experimental and comparison groups of sufficient size and representativeness to allow statistical analyses beyond the descriptive statistics reported thus far. Cause and effect relationships can be tested with quasi-experimental designs (see Murphy 1989a). Some of the studies reviewed have extensive data sets that provide an opportunity for multiple triangulation approaches (see Murphy, 1989b), but use of these approaches is limited.

Several recently published papers can guide future research in catastrophic loss. Several integrative reviews published in past volumes of *Annual Review of Nursing Research* are instructive. For example, Stevenson (1984, p. 66) in her chapter on adulthood states, "The occurrence of health problems is both an overlay upon the already complex mission of adult life and simultaneously an additional stimulus for enhancing emotional maturation. Thus, a fertile field for research and theory building is provided by the constant interplay between health crises and developmental processes." Similarly, reviews by Norbeck (1988) on social support and Roy (1988) on information-processing provide approaches to the study of mediating factors between stress and health status and adaptation.

Human responses to threatened events have relevance because of the anxiety generated by ambiguity, uncertainty, and hopelessness about future generations. Meisenhelder and LaCharite (1989) considered affective, neuro-cognitive, and physiological linkages to coping with fear of HIV.

A 1985 volume edited by Sowder for the National Institutes of Mental Health has many good suggestions for catastrophic event studies. In a recent paper, Lanza (1986) describes some characteristics of victims of international terrorism that may generate researchable issues.

Studies on the effects of catastrophic experiences on families are a neglected but important area of study. Some recent papers can guide design and analysis of family studies (Gilliss, 1983; Uphold & Strickland, 1989).

Consultation at the time of research problem development is urged. Discussions with experts early in the research process assist investigators to plan for optimal study conditions, such as sampling, instrument selection, and data collection and analysis procedures.

REFERENCES

American Psychiatric Association. (1980). *Diagnostic and statistical manual of psychiatric disorders* (3rd ed.). Washington, DC: Author.

Barrick, B. (1988). The willingness of nursing personnel to care for patients with acquired immune deficiency syndrome: A survey study and recommendations. *Journal of Professional Nursing, 4,* 366–372.

Boatright, C. J. (1985). Children as victims of disaster. In J. Laube & S. A. Murphy (Eds.), *Perspectives on disaster recovery* (pp. 131–149). Norwalk, CT: Appleton-Century-Crofts.

Bugen, L. (1977). Human grief: A model for prediction and intervention. *American Journal of Orthopsychiatry, 47,* 166–174.

Center for Disease Control. (1987). Update: Acquired immunodeficiency syndrome—United States. *MMWR, 36,* 522–527.

Cohen, F. L., Hardin, S. B., Nehring, W.,.Keough, M. A., Laurenti, S., McNabb, J., Platis, C., & Weber, C. (1988). Physical and psychosocial health status three years after catastrophic illness—botulism. *Issues in Mental Health Nursing, 9,* 387–398.

Cowan, M. E., & Murphy, S. A. (1985). Identification of postdisaster high risk bereavement predictors. *Nursing Research, 34,* 71–75.

Derogatis, L. R. (1977). *SCL-90-R: Administration, scoring and procedures manual-I.* Baltimore, MD: Clinical Psychometrics Research.

Derogatis, L. R., Lipman, R. S., Rickels, K., Uehlenhuth, E. H., & Covi, L. (1974). The Hopkins Symptom Checklist (HSCL): A self-report symptom inventory. *Behavioral Science, 19,* 1–15.

Dynes, R. R. (1970). Organizational involvement and changes in community structure in disaster. *American Behavioral Scientist, 13,* 430–439.

Gilson, B. S., Gilson, J. S., Bergner, M., Bobitt, R. A., Kressel, S., Pollard, W. E., & Vesselago, M. (1975). The Sickness Impact Profile: Development of an outcome measure of health care. *American Journal of Public Health, 65,* 1304–1310.

Gilliss, C. (1983). The family as a unit of analysis: Strategies for the nurse researcher. *Advances in Nursing Science, 5*(3), 50–59.

Glittenberg, J. (1981). Variation in stress and coping in three migrant settlements in Guatemala City. *Image: Journal of Nursing Scholarship, 13,* 243–246.

Glittenberg, J. (1985). Social upheaval and recovery in Guatemala City after the 1976 earthquake. In J. Laube & S. A. Murphy (Eds.), *Perspectives on disaster recovery* (pp. 263–281). Norwalk, CT: Appleton-Century-Crofts.

Green, B. L. (1982). Assessing levels of psychological impairment following disaster: Consideration of actual and methodological dimensions. *Journal of Nervous and Mental Disease, 170,* 544–552.

Hardin, S. B., & Cohen, F. L. (1988). Psychosocial effects of a catastrophic botulism outbreak. *Archives of Psychiatric Nursing, 2,* 173–184.

Hartsough, D. M. (1985). Measurement of the psychological effects of disaster. In J. Laube & S. A. Murphy (Eds.), *Perspectives on disaster recovery* (pp. 34–35). Norwalk, CT: Appleton-Century-Crofts.

Hawkins, N. G., Davies, R., & Holmes, T. H. (1957). Evidence of psychosocial factors in the development of pulmonary tuberculosis. *American Review of Tuberculosis and Pulmonary Disease, 75,* 768–780.

Herick, G. (1985). *Anti-gay prejudice and public relations to AIDS.* Unpublished manuscript.

Hyman, R., & Woog, P. (1982). Stressful life events and illness onset: A review of critical variables. *Research in Nursing & Health, 5,* 155–163.

Karasek, R. A. (1979). Job demands, job decison latitude, and mental strain: Implications for job redesign. *Administrative Science Quarterly, 24,* 285–308.

Kiger, J. (1984). *A reliability assessment of the SCL-90-R using a longitudinal natural disaster bereaved sample.* Unpublished master's thesis, Oregon Health Sciences University, Portland, OR.

Kiger, J., & Murphy, S. A. (1987). Reliability assessment of the SCL-90-R using a longitudinal bereaved disaster population. *Western Journal of Nursing Research, 9,* 572–588.

Kreps, G. A. (1978). The organization of disaster response: Some fundamental theoretical issues. In E. L. Quarantelli (Ed.), *Disasters: Theory and research* (pp. 65–85). Beverly Hills, CA: Sage.

Lanza, M. L. (1986). Victims of international terrorism. *Issues in Mental Health Nursing, 8,* 95–108.

LaRocco, J. M., House, J. S., & French, J. R. P. (1980). Social support, occupational stress, and health. *Journal of Health and Social Behavior, 21,* 202–218.

Laube, J. (1974). *Responses of the health care workers' family-community role conflict in disaster and the psychological consequences of resolution.* Unpublished doctoral dissertation, Texas Women's University, Austin, TX.

Laube, J. (1985). Health care providers as disaster victims. In J. Laube & S. A. Murphy (Eds.), *Perspectives on disaster recovery* (pp. 210–230). Norwalk, CT: Appleton-Century-Crofts.

Lazarus, R. S., & Folkman, S. (1984). The coping process: An alternative to traditional formulations. *Stress, appraisal, and coping* (pp. 141–180). New York: Springer Publishing Co.

Logue, J. N. (1978). *Long-term effects of a major natural disaster: The Hurricane Agnes flood in the Wyoming Valley of Pennsylvania.* Unpublished doctoral dissertation, Columbia University, NY.

Logue, J., Melick, M., & Struening, E. (1981). A study of health and mental health status following a major natural disaster. In R. Simmons (Ed.), *Research in* community mental health: An annual compilation of research, Vol. II (pp. 217–274). Greenwich, CT: JAI Press.

Lovejoy, N. C., & Moran, T. A. (1988). Selected AIDS beliefs, behaviors, and informational needs of homosexual and bisexual men with AIDS or ARC. International Journal of Nursing Studies, 25, 207–216.

Matteson, M. T., & Ivancevich, J. M. (1987). Controlling work stress. Effective human resource and management strategies (pp. 18–32). San Francisco: Jossey-Bass.

McKusick, L. (1985). AIDS and sexual behavior reported by gay men in San Francisco. American Journal of Public Health, 75, 1449–1450.

Meisenhelder, J. B., & LaCharite, C. L. (1989). Fear of contagion: A stress response to acquired immunodeficiency syndrome. Advances in Nursing Science, 11(2), 29–38.

Melick, M. E. (1976). Social, psychological and medical aspects of stress-related illness in the recovery period of a natural disaster. Unpublished doctoral dissertation, State University of New York at Albany, Albany, NY.

Melick, M. E. (1985). The health of postdisaster populations: A review of the literature. In J. Laube & S. A. Murphy (Eds.), Perspectives on disaster recovery (pp. 179–209). Norwalk, CT: Appleton-Century-Crofts.

Miles, M. S., Demi, A. S., & Mostyn-Aker, P. (1984). Rescue workers' reactions following the Hyatt Hotel disaster. Death Education, 8, 315–331.

Mitchell, J. T. (1983). When disaster strikes. . . . The critical incident stress debriefing process. Journal of Emergency Medical Services, 8(1), 36–39.

Murphy, S. A. (1982). Coping with stress following a natural disaster: The volcanic eruption of Mt. St. Helens. Dissertation Abstracts International, 42, 10B, p. 4014, (University Microfilms No. 82-07, 736)

Murphy, S. A. (1984). Stress levels and health status of victims of a natural disaster. Research in Nursing & Health, 7, 205–215.

Murphy, S. A. (1986a). Perceptions of stress, coping, and recovery one and three years after a natural disaster. Issues in Mental Health Nursing, 8, 63–77.

Murphy, S. A. (1986b). Health and recovery status of natural disaster victims one and three years later. Research in Nursing & Health, 9, 331–340.

Murphy, S. A. (1987). Self-efficacy and social support. Mediators of stress on mental health following a natural disaster. Western Journal of Nursing Research, 9, 58–86.

Murphy, S. A. (1989a). An explanatory model of recovery from disaster loss. Research in Nursing & Health, 12, 67–76.

Murphy, S. A. (1989b). Multiple triangulation. Applications in a program of nursing research. Nursing Research, 38, 294–297.

Murphy, S. A., & Stewart, B. J. (1985–1986). Linked pairs of subjects: A method for increasing the sample size in a study of bereavement. Omega, 16, 141–153.

Norbeck, J. S. (1988). Social support. In J. J. Fitzpatrick, R. L. Taunton, & J. Q. Benoliel, (Eds.), Annual Review of Nursing Research (pp. 85–109). New York: Springer Publishing Co.

Pilisuk, M., & Acredolo, C. (1988). Fear of technological hazards: One concern of many? Social Behavior, 3, 17–24.

Roy, C. (1988). Information-processing. In J. J. Fitzpatrick, R. L. Taunton, & J. Q. Benoliel, (Eds.), Annual Review of Nursing Research (pp. 237–262). New York: Springer Publishing Co.

Sarason, I., Johnson, J., & Siegel, J. (1978). Assessing the impact of life changes: Development of the life experiences survey. *Journal of Consulting and Clinical Psychology, 46,* 932–946.

Sowder, B. J. (Ed.). (1985). *Disasters and mental health: Selected contemporary perspectives.* (HHS Publication No. ADM 85-1421). Washington, DC: U.S. Government Printing Office.

Spitzer, R. L., Endicott, J., Fleiss, J., & Cohen, J. (1970). The Psychiatric Status Schedule. *Archives of General Psychiatry, 23,* 41–51.

Stanitis, M. A., & Winder, A. E. (1986). Nurses' beliefs about nuclear war avoidance. *Public Health Nursing, 3,* 264–270.

Stevenson, J. S. (1984). Adulthood: A promising focus for future research. In H. H. Werley & J. J. Fitzpatrick (Eds.), *Annual Review of Nursing Research* (pp. 55–74). New York: Springer Publishing Co.

Uphold, C. R., & Strickland, O. L. (1989). Issues related to the unit of analysis in family nursing research. *Western Journal of Nursing Research, 11,* 405–417.

U.S. Public Health Service. (1976). *Disaster assistance and emergency mental health.* (DHEW Publication No. ADM 76-327). Washington, DC: U.S. Department of Health, Education and Welfare.

U.S. Department Of Health, Education, and Welfare (1975). Public Health Service, National Center for Health Statistics, Publication in Vital and Health Statistics: Series 1, #11. *Health interview survey procedure 1957–1974,* (DHW Publication No. HRA 75-1311). Washington, DC: U.S. Government Printing Office.

Verbosky, S. J., & Ryan, D. A. (1988). Female partners of Vietnam veterans: Stress by proximity. *Issues in Mental Health Nursing, 9,* 95–104.

Wenger, D. E. (1978). Community response to disaster: Functional and structural alterations. In E. L. Quarantelli (Ed.), *Disasters: Theory and research* (pp. 17–47). Beverly Hills, CA: Sage.

Wilkinson, C. B. (1985). The psychological consequences of disasters. *Psychiatric Annals, 15,* 135, 138–139.

Williams, A. B., D'Aquila, R. T., & Williams, A. E. (1987). HIV infection in intravenous drug abusers. *Image: The Journal of Nursing Scholarship, 19,* 179–183.

Chapter 4

Family Caregiving for the Elderly

BARBARA A. GIVEN
COLLEGE OF NURSING
MICHIGAN STATE UNIVERSITY

CHARLES W. GIVEN
COLLEGE OF HUMAN MEDICINE
MICHIGAN STATE UNIVERSITY

CONTENTS

Characteristics of the Caregiver
Characteristics of the Care Recipient
The Processes of Caring for Elderly in the Home
Caregivers' Reactions to the Caregiving Processes
    Caregiver Burdens
    Positive Responses
Impact of Caregiving on Caregiver Physical Health
Impact of Caregiving on Employment and Other Roles
Formal and Informal Support and Resources
Interventions
Recommendations for Future Research

This literature review was supported through four grants, "Caregiver Responses to Managing Elderly Patients at Home," grant #1 R01 AG06584, funded by Health and Human Services National Institute on Aging, Charles W. Given, Ph.D., Principal Investigator; "Impact of Alzheimer's Disease on Family Caregivers," grant #1 R01 MH41766, funded by Health and Human Services National Institute of Mental Health, Charles W. Given, Ph.D., Principal Investigator; "Family Homecare for Cancer: A Community-Based Model," grant #1 R01 NR01915, funded by Health and Human Services National Center for Nursing Research, Barbara A. Given, Ph.D., R.N., F.A.A.N., Principal Investigator; "Family Homecare for Cancer," grant #PBR-32, funded by the American Cancer Society, Barbara A. Given, Ph.D., R.N., F.A.A.N., Principal Investigator.

Family members provide the majority of care for the disabled elderly. Until recently, relatively little has been written about the impact on the caregiver of caring for a physically dependent or cognitively impaired elder in the home. Major demographic shifts highlighted by the rapidly increasing proportion of elderly in the population have resulted in increased demand for long-term care. The importance of family and home care as a major form of long-term care has emerged as a significant social issue. Therefore, the purposes of this chapter are to: (a) review the existing literature on family caregiving, (b) describe the common themes and findings that emerge from the research, and (c) propose directions for future research.

For this review, which covers the last decade, computerized databases were used from the National Library of Medicine, including MEDLINE, health planning and administration, the Library of Congress computerized system, and AGELINE. Also, reviews of major journals from social work, marriage and the family, gerontology and geriatrics, psychology, and sociology were used to supplement the existing nursing research. Unpublished materials from current research were included when researchers made them available.

Researchers approach this topic from the perspective that caring for the elderly is difficult, time-consuming, and emotionally and physically burdensome. Once the burdens become too great, families will forego caring in favor of institutionalizing their relative. Thus, major themes in the caregiving research focus on identifying those caregivers most vulnerable to the demands of caring, those patients most difficult to care for, those tasks that are most demanding, and those support systems that provide respite from the care demands.

A review of the characteristics of caregivers will provide the initial focus of the chapter, including their relationship to the patient, their gender, and several important beliefs and attitudes that appear to influence their reactions to the caregiving situation. From caregivers, the focus will shift to describing the patients, aspects of caregiving situation, the reactions to caregiving, and the influence of formal services and informal supports on caregivers' ability to care for their elderly in the home. A brief review of the interventions to alleviate burdens of caregivers and assist caregivers to continue caring is included. This chapter concludes with recommendations for future research.

CHARACTERISTICS OF THE CAREGIVER

The common family caregiving situation involves a woman, often over 55 years old, as the primary provider of services with support primarily from other family members and, to a lesser extent, from friends and neighbors (Frankfather, Smith, & Caro, 1981; Horowitz, 1985b; Stone, Cafferata, & Sangle, 1987). One family member, who usually shares the household with the care recipient, occupies the role of primary caregiver, while other family members play secondary roles (C. W. Given & B. Given, 1988a; Soldo & Myllyluoma, 1983; Stone et al., 1987). As a consequence of the longevity of women, elderly males are cared for by spouses; whereas elderly females are cared for by children, usually daughters. In the absence of both spouse and children, siblings, grandchildren, nieces, and nephews take on caregiving (Brody, 1981; Cicerelli, 1983; C. W. Given & B. Given, 1988a, Gwyther & George, 1986; Soldo & Myllyluoma, 1983; Stone et al., 1987).

The processes through which adult children become caregivers are poorly understood. Horowitz (1985b) notes that one child is called to be a caregiver more from proximity and necessity than by choice. Treas, Gronvold, and Bengston (1980) could not confirm birth order as a determinant of caregiving and parent–child relationships. Wilson (1989a) describes the process that family members employ in deciding to become a caregiver. Caregivers engage in what she terms "recasting" of their experiences and appraisals of the relative. Once they recast, then they decide whether or not to adopt the caregiving role. According to Wilson, the decision to take on the home care of a demented relative is motivated primarily by a keen sense of moral duty.

Phillips and Rempusheski (1986) and Phillips (1983) described the dynamics of the caregiver–elder relationship and how this influenced the outcomes of caregiving. They examined the perceptions of the history of events, the "quality" of family caregiving, and how taking on the caregiving role changed other roles and created interpersonal strains, possibly leading to abuse of the patient. Motenko (1989) found that frustrations and gratifications of the caregiver were important in the success of caregiving arrangements. Archbold, Stewart, Greenlick, and Harvath, (1990) explored the extent to which caregivers believed they were prepared to assume the caregiving role. From this, Archbold et al. (1990) defined a concept that they labeled "preparedness." Haley, Levine, Brown, and Bartolucci (1987) and Lawton, Kleban, Moss, Rovine, and Glicksman (1989) defined similar concepts related to the caregivers' abilities to assume and master the physical, social, and psychological demands of caring for an elderly person in the home.

A number of researchers have examined the relationship between the gender of spouse caregivers and their reported levels of burden and depression. Those studies that controlled for any differences in the physical or cognitive functioning of the patient found few if any differences in reported levels of caregiver burden according to the gender of the caregiver (Fitting, Rabins, Lucas, & Eastham, 1986; Johnson, 1983; Miller, 1987; Pruchno &

Resch, 1989; S. H. Zarit, Todd, & J. M. Zarit, 1986). Some researchers found that wife caregivers report poorer mental and physical health than husband caregivers (Fitting et al., 1986; Miller, 1987). Several investigators (Pruchno & Resch, 1989; M. P. Quayhagen & M. Quayhagen, 1988; Young & Kahana, 1989) suggested that wives and daughters express more caregiv-ing-related burdens than husbands. A number of theories have been proposed to explain these differences, including mechanisms for maintaining control (Miller, 1987; Pagel, Becker, & Coppel, 1985) and social supports (Barusch & Spaid, 1989). There are few consistent findings in response to caregiving based on gender differences.

Three factors lead to assumption of the caregiving role: demographic imperatives (i.e., only child or only female child), geographic obligations of reciprocity, and situational factors (i.e., child with the least valued competing commitments). Further research is needed to focus on the demographic and family dynamics that lead to the selection of the family member to adopt the caregiving role when a spouse is unavailable.

CHARACTERISTICS OF THE CARE RECIPIENT

Functional or mental status of the patient, such as, immobility, incontinence, behavioral and cognitive problems, as well as physical and emotional health status have emerged as important factors contributing to patterns and con-sequences of family care (Branch & Jette, 1983; Horowitz, 1985a). Research on characteristics of persons being cared for in-home have focused on: dependencies in self-care activities, mobility, and instrumental activities of daily living (Branch & Jette, 1983; Horowitz, 1985a), cognitive status, and behavioral problems (Deimling & Bass, 1986). Several authors have ex-amined the interactions of the dependencies (Haley & Pardo, 1989; Pearson, Verma, & Nellett, 1988; Teri, Borson, Kiyak, & Yamagishi, 1989). Stetz (1987) and Stetz and Johnson (1989) have examined how dependencies in activities of daily living (ADL), instrumental activities of daily living (IADL), and cognitive impairments translate into involvement in care for the caregiver. Other studies have focused on how the cognitive and behavioral manifestations affect caregiver burdens and mental health status of those caring for persons with Alzheimer's disease and related dementias (Burke, Houston, Boust, & Roccaforte, 1989; Mace, 1986; Moritz, Kasl, & Berk-man, 1989; Noelker & Poulshock, 1982; Pruchno & Resch, 1989; S. H. Zarit & J. M. Zarit, 1982).

There is a debate in the literature regarding whether the physical or mental impairment of the patient makes managing the care more difficult for caregivers (Mace, 1986; Montgomery, Gonyea, & Hooyman, 1985; Noelker & Poulshock, 1982; Rabins, Mace, & Lucas, 1982; B. Robinson, 1983). In some instances, patients may be "able" to perform tasks but, because of normative prescriptions or cultural values, not engage in these tasks. In other situations patients may not be able to perform or even to assist with the tasks.

In the caregiving literature, patients are characterized according to gender, relationship to the caregiver, marital status, the numbers of dependencies in ADL and IADL, their cognitive status and, less frequently, according to the diagnoses assigned to them by health care providers (Stoller & Earl, 1983). Research is needed to describe how patient deficits are identified and then compare how family members' interpretations of those needs are translated into care tasks. Minimum criteria and standards for assessing the quality of care delivered by family to dependent individuals could then be developed. More information and description is needed about characteristics of the care recipient and how they influence the overall caregiving process.

THE PROCESSES OF CARING FOR ELDERLY IN THE HOME

Studies of the caregiving process generally focus on the specific tasks of care most often defined in terms of performance or assistance with the activities of daily living and the instrumental activities related to cooking, cleaning/ laundry, transportation, and management of finances. Caregiving can then be described in relation to which tasks are completed, by whom, how often, and with what result (Archbold et al., 1990; Cicerelli, 1983; Clark & Rakowski, 1983; C. W. Given, Stommel et al., 1988; Robinson & Thurnher, 1979; Stoller & Earl, 1983). Focusing on the tasks of caregiving directs attention away from the planning, organizing, monitoring, and supervising processes that caregivers must complete. These indirect care activities may engender stress, and in some regards, may be more demanding than direct care activities (Bowers, 1987; Stetz, 1987).

The specific combination of functional limitations and cognitive impairments dictate the nature and time demands of caregiving tasks. Physical assistance may be discrete and amenable to planning and scheduling, and while caring for a person with dementia may be less physically demanding, it also may include substantial supervision, loss of sleep, or loss of companionship. Caregiving tasks range from occasional errands to 24-hour care (Archbold, 1980; Archbold et al., 1990; C. W. Given, Stommel et al., 1988; Lang & Brody, 1983; Silliman & Sternberg, 1988; Stetz, 1987). Involvement in caregiving may vary with the extent to which the elderly person is able to adapt to physical impairments, is willing to do certain activities, and has cognitive skills related to organizing and executing the tasks. In addition, the ability of the caregiver to detect the need for assistance and the long-standing nature of the role relationships between caregiver and patient may affect caregiving (C. W. Given & B. Given, 1989; C. W. Given, Stommel et al., 1988; Horowitz, 1985a; Lang & Brody, 1983; Stone et al., 1987).

The description of tasks of care has been organized in different ways. These include organizing caregiving tasks according to whether the caregiver carries out the tasks (care provider) or manages their performance by employing others to carry out the direct tasks (Archbold, 1983; Archbold et al., 1990) according to the level of intensity (weekly to daily) (B. Given & C. W. Given, 1989), according to the degree of intimacy involved (Horowitz, 1985b), and according to the demands of care assigned by the caregiver (Bowers, 1987; Phillips, 1983; Phillips & Rempusheski, 1985, 1986; Rempusheski & Phillips, 1988; Stetz, 1987; Stetz & Hanson, 1989; Stetz & Johnson, 1989).

Caregivers who spend time and energy with direct physical and personal care may find tasks restrictive and confining. Disruption of domestic routines and decreased personal, social, and recreational time become pervasive problems for family caregivers (Frankfather et al., 1981; Horowitz, 1985b; Rabins et al., 1982). Horowitz (1985b) categorizes these activities into a hierarchy of instrumental assistance, the tasks that require intermittent basic help, the in-home assistances (meal preparation, etc.), which are the more labor-intensive services requiring regular time commitments, and the more intensive and intimate personal and health care services. The more personal care is most frequently provided by those caregivers who are most closely related to the care recipient. Information and research on the caregiver role as manager or mediator with formal organizations and agencies is limited, and no systematic investigations could be found.

In a grounded theory approach, Bowers (1987) conceptualized the organization of caregiving as the "meaning or purpose a caregiver attributes to an activity" (p. 21.) She described both observable and nonobservable processes, including emotional support, planning, and decision-making. Bowers identified five dimensions of the process of family caregiving: instrumental; anticipatory; preventive, which includes monitoring; supervisory, which includes arrangements; and protective care activities. In her conceptualization, only instrumental activity included the traditionally described hands-on care.

Stetz (1987) classified the tasks of caring according to the demands they imposed on spouse caregivers of adult cancer patients. The most frequent demands were managing physical care, treatment and changes in treatment, household and financial responsibilities, alterations in caregiver well-being and patterns in living, constant vigilance, unmet needs with the health care system, cancer itself, anticipating the future, and altering relationship with an ill spouse. These categories of demands included direct care activities, but also were congruent with the anticipatory, supervisory, and protective categories suggested by Bowers (1987).

Work by Collins, B. Given, and C. W. Given (1988), and C. W. Given, B. Given, and Ogle (1988) demonstrates why the focus on tasks alone does not adequately capture the dynamics and intensity of the family care role. Anticipation, prevention, supervision, and protection require observations and judgments at a more complex and sophisticated level and await empirical confirmation.

In assessing the processes of caregiving, researchers must consider the natural course of the caregiving trajectory and the point in that course where the assessment is being made. Literature describing differences in such processes across a longitudinal care trajectory is unavailable. To date researchers have not examined the congruence between what caregivers do and what care recipients really need. The conceptualizations by Bowers (1987), Stetz and Hanson (1989), and Wilson (1989a) are important perspectives that broaden the process of caregiving beyond a set of tasks.

The process or natural course of caregiving has not been examined. Knowledge about the acquisition of caregiving skills is limited, as is knowledge about the changes in processes of care across time and how preparedness alters the caregivers' reactions. Attention to how the processes of care vary as caregivers become more accustomed to the role, master the tasks, and adapt to the caregiving role is also absent. There are very few longitudinal studies in which investigators describe the process of caregiving by family members. Archbold et al. (1990) have used the concept of preparedness. Lawton, Kleban, et al. (1989) have developed a subscale that referred to caregiving mastery. However, neither concept has been described adequately or been employed in longitudinal studies to determine how caregivers change in their reactions as they become more prepared or master the tasks and demands of caregiving.

CAREGIVERS' REACTIONS TO THE CAREGIVING PROCESSES

Most of the research on family caregivers has been focused on reactions of caregivers to their caregiving role and the caregiving processes. Reactions to caring have been both positive and negative. However, most research has been focused on the negative impact that caregiving has imposed on family members (Blank, Atwood, & Longman, 1989; Chenowith & Spencer, 1986; B. Given, King, Collins, & C. W. Given, 1988; Krause, 1987; S. H. Zarit et al. 1986). The concept of caregiver burden (strain) has been defined as the persistent hardships, stress, reactions of caring, or as the physical and psychological, financial, and social problems experienced by family members providing care in the home (Cohen & Eisdorfer, 1988; Kosberg & Cairl, 1986; McCorkle et al. 1989; Montgomery et al., 1985; Noelker & Bass, 1989; Oberst & James, 1985; Pearson et al., 1988; S. H. Zarit & J. M. Zarit, 1982). Caregiver burden has been biopsychosocial reaction of the primary caregiver resulting from an imbalance of demands relative to resources available.

Caregiver Burdens

Montgomery et al. (1985) divided burdens into objective and subjective components. Archbold and Stewart (1990), building on the work of Montgomery et al. (1985), measured eleven components of caregiver strain that included strain from direct care, managed care, caregiving role expectations, communication, lack of resources, economic burden, tension in relationship, manipulation, role conflict, and global strain. S. H. Zarit, Reever, and Bach-Peterson (1980) developed a unidimensional scale to measure caregiver burdens. Poulshock and Deimling (1984) and Lawton, Brody, and Saperstein (1989), using factor analytic techniques, identified multidimensional scales to measure burden. Gwyther and George (1986) employed a multidimensional, well-being scale to measure caregivers' reactions over a 6-month period. Poulshock and Deimling (1984) included a measure of caregiver depression as did Moritz, Kasl, and Berkman (1989), Schulz, Tompkins, and Rau (1990), and Stommel, C. W. Given, and B. Given (1990). However, in order to identify the amount of depression associated with caregiving, it is essential to compare persons experiencing caregiving with age, sex, and occupation-matched groups who are in caregiving situations.

Researchers have found that caregiving restricted family members' social lives and their interactions with other family members (Moritz et al., 1989; Shapiro & Tuti, 1988; Stetz, 1987). Caregiving also imposed a heavy psychologic impact on the caregiver, whether viewed as depression, decreased satisfaction or lowered well-being (Gwyther & George, 1986; Kosberg & Cairl, 1986; Oberst & Scott, 1988; Pearson et al., 1988; B. Robinson, 1983; Worcester & M. P. Quayhagen, 1983). Although findings were inconsistent, involvement in self-care tasks, hours of care required per day, and the amount of supervision required have been related to the burdens of caregiving (Deimling & Bass, 1986; Gwyther & George, 1986; Kiecolt-Glaser et al., 1987; Montgomery et al., 1985; Moritz et al., 1989; Stommel et al., 1990).

In general, as more time was devoted to caregiving and as the tasks became more intimate, caregivers were less able to control timing of tasks, and thus, experienced greater burdens (Archbold, 1983; Archbold et al., 1990; Cicerelli, 1983; Montgomery et al., 1985). Wilson (1989b) and Stetz and Hanson (1989) reported that the pervasive sense of not knowing what to expect or how to interpret what was happening—the fear of the unknown—both in terms of what was happening to the patient, as well as the open ended nature of the caring process, led to increased strain among caregivers.

The theoretical and empirical utility of a caregiver burden concept remains controversial. Recent reviewers of this construct (Montgomery et al., 1985; Vitaliano, 1988) attempted to evaluate the role of burden in caregiving research. Vitaliano equated burden with distress. In Vitaliano's approach, distress was the quotient resulting when the exposure to stressor plus vulnerability were divided by the amount of psychological and social resources. Montgomery (1989) and Stommel et al. (1990) presented a summary of findings related to caregiver burdens and the more general mental health parameter of depression. Future research is needed to clarify the role of caregiver burden and general mental health status.

Positive Responses

Positive aspects of caregiving, although not as well documented (Archbold et al., 1990; Gwyther & George, 1986; Lawton, Kleban et al., 1989), are important for a comprehensive view of caregiving. Positive feelings about caregiving have emerged as significant predictors of less stressful caregiving experiences (Cantor, 1983; Cicerelli, 1983; Gwyther & George, 1986; Horowitz, 1985b; B. Robinson, 1983). Positive aspects of care primarily include a caregiver's feeling of self-satisfaction, gratification, and increased self-respect stemming from the knowledge that one is fulfilling a valued responsibility successfully and coping with a personal challenge (Archbold et al., 1990; Collins, C. W. Given, B. Given, & King, 1988; Horowitz, 1985a; Motenko, 1989; Reece, Walz, & Hageboeck, 1983).

Hirshfield (1983) described caregiver behaviors based on feelings of mutuality and recognition by caregivers that they received as much from the caregiving relationship as thay had given to patient care. If mutuality existed, caregivers viewed themselves as engaging in an important and useful social role. Archbold et al. (1990) took the idea of mutality further as they identified a concept labeled "rewards of caregiving." Rewards of caregiving were related to the caregiver's abilities to ascribe meaning and value to their own care situation. Mutuality and rewards buffered caregiver strain resulting from feelings of obligation and resentment (Horowitz, 1985a; Phillips & Rempusheski, 1985, 1986). Increased self-esteem came from feelings of competence, fulfillment of fundamental social roles, and meeting basic, affective familial obligations (Archbold et al., 1990; Collins & C. W. Given, 1988; B. Given et al., 1988; Phillips, 1983; Wellisch, Landsverk, Guidera, Pasnau, & Fawzy, 1983).

A promising approach toward understanding caregiving is to describe and classify the natural course of the caregiver experience. Oberst (1989) has proposed a model to examine the relationship between coping strategies and caregiver burden and well-being on a longitudinal basis. Archbold et al. (1990), in a longitudinal study, reported that the number of tasks increased over time and that there was an associated increase in confinement and caregiver global strain. McCorkle et al. (1989) found that in spouse caregivers of patients with lung cancer, when death occurred, improvement in well-being over time was higher in those spouses who had assistance from clinical nurse specialists.

Without longitudinal data it is difficult to understand how, or under what circumstances, some caregivers adjust to caregiving and perceive fewer burdens, whereas others perceive greater burdens over time. In an attempt to explain variations in perceived burdens, researchers have examined variations in the social supports, the amount of assistance received from family and friends, and the amount of services provided by formal agencies available to the caregiver, especially among family members involved in similar caregiving processes.

IMPACT OF CAREGIVING ON CAREGIVER PHYSICAL HEALTH

Although several researchers have focused on psychosocial effects of caregiving, focus on the effects on physical health status of caregivers is limited. The caregiver, when faced with dwindling resources of energy, time, and money, may be forced to choose between self-care or the care needs of the dependent elderly, and their own health status may deteriorate (Bunting, 1989). Kiecolt-Glaser and Glaser (1989) and Vitaliano (1988) examined the impact of caregiving on the immune system of the caregiver. Gwyther and George (1986) addressed physical health status through self reports. Stommel et al. (1990) and B. Given and C. W. Given (1989) suggested that measures often used to determine the physical health of the caregiver may be confounded by depression or negative reaction to care.

Wilson (1989b), and Smallegan (1985) argue that when caregivers' physical and emotional well-being are eroded, caregivers change perspectives about care and may decide to institutionalize the relative. It is important to understand the relationship between physical health of the caregiver and his or her response to care as well as the impact on the care recipient. Thus, while caregivers, particularly elderly spouses, reported that caregiving had caused their health to deteriorate, little objective confirmation exists in the literature (Satariano, Minkler, & Langhauser, 1984; Stetz, 1987; Yankelovich, Skelley, & White, 1986). It is important that the effect of caregiving on the incidence of exacerbations of existing chronic conditions and the onset of new physical problems among caregivers be documented.

IMPACT OF CAREGIVING ON EMPLOYMENT AND OTHER ROLES

Evidence regarding the impact of caregiving on ability of families to carry out work roles is conflicting. Among adult daughters, responsibilities to parents may take precedence over responsibilities to spouse, children, or others because care of parents is seen as the most pressing need (Horowitz, 1985b; Noelker & Poulshock, 1982; Rabins et al., 1982). Missing from nursing and other literature, except in the work of Brody and Schoonover (Brody, 1985; Brody & Schoonover, 1986), is a clear articulation of how other competing role demands impinge on the caregiving process. Caregivers with other responsibilities, including those who work outside the home, are reported to experience inhibition, disruption, and withdrawal from work role involvement (B. Given & C. W. Given, 1989; C. W. Given & B. Given, 1989; Horowitz, 1985a; Stone et al., 1987; Vess, Moreland, & Schwebel, 1985). Adult children who exercise multiple roles, including working, may be more burdened. However, employment or other roles outside of the family may be key to caregiver well-being (Barnes, C. W. Given, & B. Given, 1990; Brody & Schoonover, 1986; Stoller & Pugliesi, 1989).

FORMAL AND INFORMAL SUPPORT AND RESOURCES

Families caring for the elderly draw on formal and informal resources for assistance. However, the family continues to provide the major portion of care. Formal care services include community agencies and the health care system. Informal support to the primary caregiver includes the assistance from other family members, relatives, and friends (Baille, Norbeck, & Barnes, 1988; Lyles, King, & B. Given, 1990; Noelker & Wallace, 1985;

M. P. Quayhagen & M. Quayhagen, 1988; Stone et al., 1987; Tennestedt, McKinley, & Sullivan, 1989).

Social support has been the most frequently studied variable that mediates stress in the caregiving situation. (Baille et al., 1988; Fiore, Coppel, Becker, & Cox, 1986; Krause, 1987; M. P. Quayhagen & M. Quayhagen, 1988). Gwyther and George (1986) found that caregivers reported poorer mental health and had lower social participation than similarly aged peers with no caregiving responsibilities. In a study of caregivers of family members with Alzheimer's disease, Scott, Roberto, and Hutton (1986) found that family support was related positively to coping effectiveness and reduced burdens. Gilhooly (1984), Fiore et al., (1986), Baille et al. (1988), and S. H. Zarit et al. (1986) found that satisfaction with the help from relatives had a positive correlation with caregiver mental health (depression). Krause (1987) reported that social support may provide a buffer from stress by increasing internal beliefs that one is cared about. Krause cautioned that thresholds exist in which social support may move from being of assistance to becoming a stressor.

Family caregivers tended to be very selective in their formal service requests (Collins, Stommel, Thiele, C. W. Given, & King, 1989; Horowitz, 1985a; Sager, 1983). Bass and Noelker (1987), Noelker and Bass (1989), and Romeis (1989) suggested that caregiver perception of the elders' needs relative to their own available resources (income and family assistance) affected the contact with the community agency. Male caregivers appeared to receive more assistance from formal caregivers than female caregivers (Johnson, 1983; Pratt, Schmall, Wright, & Cleland, 1985; S. H. Zarit et al., 1986). Utilization of community services was low especially for patients with cognitive deficits (Birkel & Jones, 1989; Yankelovich et al., 1986). Oberst (1989) suggested that optimism may have influenced appraisal of needs and the decision to seek social support. Formal support and respite programs may have affected caregiver physical health positively (M. P. Quayhagen & M. Quayhagen, 1988) but may not have reduced caregiver burdens (Archbold, 1983; National Long Term Care Channelling Demonstration, 1986; Weissert, Cready, & Pawelak, 1988).

Formal services may not reduce burdens because families use agencies to assist in caregiving only as a last resort (Chappell & Guse, 1989). Methodologic issues, in part, may account for the weak relationships observed between formal service use and caregiver burden. Information on the use and value of formal community agencies is difficult to ascertain and has not been investigated carefully. Recall of service use may be an issue. Locating services and accessing them appears to be a significant barrier to use, and the intricate procedures governing eligibility and third party reimbursement discourage use of formal services under all but desperate circumstances.

The social class of the caregiver tends not to affect the amount of help given as much as it affects the type of assistance (Archbold, 1983). The amount of assistance provided does little to buffer the stress experienced by the primary caregiver (C. W. Given, B. Given, & Ogle, 1988; Horowitz, 1985a; Noelker & Poulshock, 1982). The perception of support emerges as a critical variable for predicting lower levels of burden or distress (Archbold, 1983; Lyles et al., 1990; Noelker & Poulshock, 1982; Stommel et al., 1990). A caregiver feeling secure that support is available if needed may carry on in the caregiving role with less stress, regardless of whether that help is ever activated. However, Oberst (1989) points out that the literature includes discussion of the consequences of receiving social support, but little attention has been directed toward the consequences of providing support.

Future researchers should examine how family caregivers reallocate their time when others provide assistance with care. Does assistance simply free them to engage in other tasks that have been abandoned because of the exigencies of caregiving? Is assistance substitutive or complementary to the tasks the caregivers provide to the family member? Does assistance from others provide any tangible or emotional respite or merely complement their care? The impact of such assistance may be examined through reported intervention studies.

INTERVENTIONS

Surprisingly little information is available about intervention programs that are supportive to families. Family caregivers often find themselves providing technical assistance and skilled home health care for which they have little prior experience (Archbold et al., 1990).

Caregiver interventions that have been studied include: caregiver education and training groups, self-help groups, comprehensive service programs (Biegel, Shore, & Gordon, 1984), and family counseling or therapy. M. P. Quayhagen and M. Quayhagen (1989), Archbold et al. (1990), Archbold (1983), Baldwin (1988), and McCorkle et al. (1989) have all implemented nursing intervention programs to assist family caregivers.

Education and training programs provide caregivers with increased knowledge concerning the aging process, information on services for older persons, and effective skills for caregiving. The programs are based on the premise that increased knowledge, information, and skills will increase caregiver competence and eliminate excess burden and distress (Biegel et al., 1984). A few investigators have tested the impact of social support, assistance, and respite care on caregiver outcomes including affective responses and reported burdens (Couper & Sheehan, 1987; Kahan, Kemp, Staples, & Brummel-Smith, 1985; Lawton, Brody, & Saperstein, 1989; Pinkston & Linsk, 1984; Priddy & Gallagher, 1985). K. M. Robinson (1988) proposed a model for family caregiving that links social skills and caregiver burden. She posited that caregivers with high social skills would be able to mobilize social support in the environment more effectively, resulting in decreased caregiver burden.

Interventions have not demonstrated significant impacts on caregivers' behaviors or beliefs or caregivers' responses to care. Similarly, self-help, coping strategies, and mutual support groups vary widely with respect to their overall purpose (information, advocacy, respite, or emotional support), membership composition, and level of activity (Baldwin, 1988; Biegel et al., 1984) and have not proven successful.

M. P. Quayhagen and M. Quayhagen (1988) used a stress-adaptation framework to examine how deterioration among Alzheimer's disease patients influences caregivers' well-being and how the declining patient condition is mediated by coping and managing strategies and support resources of the caregivers. The coping strategies used were help-seeking, problem-solving, and existential and were associated with caregiver well-being. Montgomery, Gonyea, and Hooyman (1985), in a large-scale study providing several types of service interventions to family members with a frail elder (half of whom were cognitively impaired), concluded that families did not come for services until they were desperate.

Mohide, Torrance, Streiner, Pringle, and Gilbert (1988) used an experimental design to offer in-home nursing care, support groups, and out-of-home respite care. They reported multiple barriers to the actual conduct of experimental interventions with patients with Alzheimer's Disease and their families. The effect of the carefully implemented 6 month intervention was disappointing in that there was little benefit to the caregiver (Mohide et al., 1988). In a longitudinal, randomized clinical trial, McCorkle et al. (1989) demonstrated that care provided by nurse specialists to family caregivers during their relatives' terminal illness improves the quality of life and well-being of the caregiver following the death of the family member.

The answer to which community services are helpful at particular points in the patients' decline to have a positive impact on caregivers' reactions, burdens, and caregivers health outcomes awaits further investigation (Office of Technology Assessment, 1987). There is little in the published literature to suggest how intervention programs "should" be organized and tailored to fit the caregiving situation. Descriptions elaborating the core content of activities for caregivers, patterns or combinations of education and support, and "crucial transition time" in the caregiving trajectory for education and support intervention are needed.

Furthermore, interventions addressing the changing needs of the caregiving situation or patient status changes across the care trajectory need to be designed (Schulz, Biegel, Morycz, & Visintainer, 1989). Caregiving interventions need to be dynamic and responsive as the family moves through multiple transitions characterized by periods of uncertainty, role changes, emotional changes, and varying care demands. Interventions for caregivers are more likely to succeed if they are tailored to caregiver knowledge and beliefs about expected outcome and caregiver ability to carry out needed care behaviors. Subjects' evaluations of the intervention, including their overall satisfaction and ratings of what aspects of the treatment they found helpful, should also be described (S. H. Zarit, 1989).

Researchers' failure to include specific assessments of conflict in the family dynamic stands in contrast to many descriptive accounts of the caregiving experience presented by a number of authors (Kuypers & Bengston, 1983; Silverstone & Hyman, 1982; Springer & Brubaker, 1984). Future caregiving studies need to elaborate on how interpersonal conflict and caregivers' appraisals and expectations operate within the caregiving situation. Other issues that need to be examined are the source of conflict between the caregiver and the elder, the influence of other family members in increasing or alleviating conflict, and the influence of increasing levels of functional or mental dependence on the quality of the relationship between the elder and caregiver. The differences among caregivers' reactions to the care recipients' physical or mental dependence also require examination. (Archbold et al., 1990; Phillips & Rempusheski, 1985, Sheehan & Nuttall, 1988).

Gallagher (1985) reviewed both the conceptual frames of reference and the strategies used to improve the outcomes of caregiving. Interventions designed to reduce caregiver burden included psychotherapeutic and self and mutual help. Major problems in implementing and testing interventions focused on identifying those most in need and those most likely to benefit from interventions. Frequently, those who are most in need may be less likely to benefit because the needs are too great and patients may be too seriously ill. Unless these differences are controlled it is difficult to test the benefits of interventions to assist family caregivers.

S. H. Zarit (1989) reviewed methodologic and design-related issues around caregiver interventions. He points to the importance of using carefully controlled designs and examining the entry criteria for sampling caregivers and patients and the mediating variables that might influence the effectiveness of the interventions. At this point, researchers have not identified caregivers most likely to respond to interventions, which interventions will be more effective, and what are the more sensitive outcome variables.

RECOMMENDATIONS FOR FUTURE RESEARCH

Current research on family caregiving for the elderly has focused on one or more of the following questions: (a) Which caregiver or patient characteristics appear to be most significant in predicting negative outcomes? (b) How do (can) families and formal agencies assist caregivers to provide care? (c) Does such assistance reduce negative responses toward caregiving or reduce negative outcomes?

Although the questions posed have been straightforward, the answers reflect the durability and complexity of the family as a major social institution. Current research has produced useful measures of caregiver burden and involvement in caregiving and has identified important gender distinctions in caregiving. Research also indicates that formal services are not widely used by caregivers.

With this information as a background, future research should consider linking the demographic, social, psychological, and network theories to the natural course of the loss of function and need for assistance. The inception of caregiving can be sudden, as with those with residual handicaps following a stroke or trauma, or occur very gradually, as with those experiencing dementing illnesses or the gradual loss of functioning due to chronic illness (Manton, 1990). Against this backdrop of the natural course of loss of function and the increasing need for assistance lie the research questions that will allow us to understand better the role of families in long-term care, and their needs for outside assistance, as well as how to deliver more effective rehabilitative and maintenance interventions for the elderly residing in the community.

More attention needs to be given to how families make decisions about the long-term care of family members and how the contexts in which these decisions are made may influence the outcome. No research on family decision-making was found. For example, elderly family members whose physical or mental health deteriorates slowly may lead to a different caregiving arrangement than when deterioration occurs suddenly and irrevocably. Virtually all research examined for this review included caregivers who had been providing assistance for varying lengths of time to elderly family members who, we must assume, experienced different courses of illness leading to varying need for assistance. Inception cohort studies of caregivers and elderly family members are needed.

Inception cohort studies would control for variations in the onset of caregiving and previous history of caring by the primary caregiver, as well as examine variations in caregivers' reactions to caring and the manner in which they engage other informal and formal assistance. Such designs would help to control for variations currently thought to be important contextual factors. Second, the testing of home care interventions using randomized clinical trials would benefit from enrolling families at the inception of caregiving. Such a design would eliminate much uncontrolled variation and would permit stratification among those variables thought to be especially important in explaining the targeted outcomes.

A second important area of research that has not been examined is the quality of the home care provided by family members. For example, to what extent does home care facilitate or hinder recovery of function or successful adaptation to impairments experienced by the elderly? Addressing such questions would require examination of the prior and current relationships between caregiver and patient and exclusion of those in which the caregiver, patient or both are depressed, or where dysfunctional relationships exist.

Once a healthy patient–caregiver relationship is established it would be possible to determine if caregivers could implement simple rehabilitation and therapeutic protocols. To date, research has examined only custodial caring influences. Is it possible that rehabilitative caring might not only have benefits for the patient but also for the caregiver who would believe that he or she may actually be helping the patient to become more independent? Loss of control over the patient's status and the inability to influence outcomes often lead to caregiver depression. More effort needs to be devoted toward involving families in rehabilitative strategies (Schulz et al., 1989).

With national attention being drawn toward the outcomes of formal care it seems eminently appropriate also to examine the outcomes of home care. What roles do families currently assume in caring: What roles might they assume? Will it be possible to transfer the technology of health maintenance and rehabilitation to the family caregiver? This will depend heavily on creating new alliances between health professions, acute care and rehabilitation settings, and the family and the home. Research in these areas holds considerable promise for containing costs and improving or preventing deterioration in patient outcome health states for extended periods.

Third, accompanying more comprehensive design and measure, is the need for the development and testing of multidimensional conceptual frames of reference that incorporate indicators of adjustment to caregiving contextual and mediating variables, and adaptation to caregiving, as well as the burdens and conflicts.

Up to the current time, research on family caregiving has been focused on the family caregiver, the impact on the caregiver, and the decision to forego caregiving in favor of long-term care that may drain public resources. The quality and appropriateness of home care provided to the care recipient as well as the caregiver needs to become the focus of future research. Standards of care based on function, self-care deficits, and cognitive status could, perhaps, reduce premature dependencies and maintain patient cognition for longer periods. Families made aware of the impact of their actions and the manner in which they could preserve patient function and cognition could implement care in accordance with such standards. At this time, there is little evidence to support that families know how to implement care effectively.

In conclusion, we urge future investigators to adopt methodologic approaches that incorporate inception cohorts of family caregivers and their patients. Identifying the point at which concern, visiting and "helping out" become transformed into "caregiving" is not always easy. However, clearer definitions can be formulated and tested. Nursing research in family caregiving is recent. The conceptual models by the nurse researchers such as Wilson (1989a; 1989b), Archbold (1980), and Bowers (1987) and the research of C. W. Given and B. Given (1988a), B. Given et al. (1988), C. W. Given, Collins, and B. Given (1988a), and Oberst (1989) are major contributions to the literature. The strength of this work is the provision of a framework within which to organize the inquiry and the findings.

Future research endeavors should be focused on the experienced, dynamic analysis of the caregiver and patients' lives including the transition into the caregiver and care recipient roles. This work is needed to meet the challenge of developing knowledge to provide quality of care and maintain the quality of lives for our aging population. Nurse researchers can do much to respond to this challenge.

ACKNOWLEDGMENTS

Special thanks go to the research team: Dr. Clare Collins, Dr. Manfred Stommel, and Dr. Sharon King, who challenge us to know the caregiving issues.

REFERENCES

Archbold, P. G. (1980). Impact of parent caring on middle-aged offspring. *Journal of Gerontological Nursing, 6*(2), 78–85.
Archbold, P. G. (1983). Impact of parent-caring on women. *Family Relations, 32,* 39–45.
Archbold, P., Stewart, B., Greenlick, M., & Harvath, T. (1990). Mutuality and preparedness as predictors of caregiver role strain. *Research in Nursing & Health, 13,* 375–384.
Baille, V., Norbeck, J., & Barnes, L. (1988). Stress, social support, and psychological stress of family caregiving of the elderly. *Nursing Research, 37,* 217–222.

Baldwin, B. A. (1988). The stress of caring: Issues confronting mid-life caregivers. *Caring, 7,* 16–18, 66.

Barnes, C. L., Given, C. W., & Given, B. (1990). *Parent caregivers: A comparison of working and non-working daughters.* Paper presented at the Conference on Human Development, Virginia Commonwealth University, Richmond, VA.

Barusch, A. S., & Spaid, W. M. (1989). Gender differences in caregiving: Why do wives report greater burden? *The Gerontologist, 29,* 667–676.

Bass, D. M., & Noelker, L. S., (1987). The influence of family caregivers on elders use of in-home services: An expanded conceptual framework. *Journal of Health and Social Behavior, 28,* 184–196.

Biegel, D., Shore, B., & Gordon, E. (1984). *Building support networks for the elderly: Theory and application.* Beverly Hills, CA: Sage.

Birkel, R. C., & Jones, C. J. (1989). A comparison of the caregiving networks of dependent elderly individuals who are lucid and those who are demented. *The Gerontologist, 29,* 114–119.

Blank, J., Atwood, J., & Longman, A. (1989). Perceived home care needs of cancer patients and their caregivers. *Cancer Nursing, 12,* 78–84.

Bowers, B. J. (1987). Intergenerational caregiving: Adult caregivers and their aging parents. *Advances in Nursing Science, 9*(2), 20–31.

Branch, L. G., & Jette, A. M. (1983). Elders' use of informal long-term care assistance. *The Gerontologist, 23,* 51–56.

Brody, E. M. (1981). Women in the middle and family help to older people. *The Gerontologist, 21*(5), 471–481.

Brody, E. M. (1985). Parent care as a normative family stress. *The Gerontologist, 25,* 19–29.

Brody, E. M., & Schoonover, C. B. (1986). Patterns of parent–care when adult daughters work and when they do not. *The Gerontologist, 26,* 372–381.

Bunting, S. M. (1989). Stress on caregivers of the elderly. *Advances in Nursing Science, 11*(2), 63–73.

Burke, W. J., Houston, M. J., Boust, S. J., & Roccaforte, W. H. (1989). Use of the geriatric depression scale in dementia of the Alzheimer's type. *Journal of American Geriatric Society, 37,* 856–860.

Cantor, M. H. (1983). Strain among caregivers: A study of experience in the U.S. *The Gerontologist, 23,* 597–604.

Chappell, N., & Guse, L. (1989). Linkages between informal and formal support. In K. S. Markides & C. L. Cooper (Eds.), *Aging, stress, and health* (pp. 219–237). New York: Wiley.

Chenowith, B., & Spencer, B. (1986). Dementia: The experience of family caregivers. *The Gerontologist, 26,* 267–272.

Cicerelli, V. (1983). Adult children and their elderly parents. In T. Brubaker (Ed.), *Family relationships in later life* (pp. 31–46). Beverly Hills, CA: Sage.

Clark, N. M., & Rakowski, W. (1983). Family caregivers of older adults: Improving helping skills. *The Gerontologist, 23,* 637–642.

Cohen, D., & Eisdorfer, C. (1988). Depression in family members caring for a relative with Alzheimer's disease. *Journal of the American Geriatric Society, 36,* 885–889.

Collins, C., & Given, C. W. (1988, November). *Use of community services among family caregivers of Alzheimer's patients.* Paper presented for the Department of Mental Health, Alzheimer's Demonstration Projects, Lansing, MI.

Collins, C., Given, B., & Given, C. W. (1988). *Impact of Alzheimer's Disease on family caregivers* (Grant #2 R01 MH41766). Rockville, MD: DHHS National Institute of Mental Health.

Collins, C., Given, C. W., Given, B., & King, S. (1988, November) *Predicting depression and positive well-being in family caregivers.* Paper presented at the 41st Annual Scientific Meeting of the Gerontological Society of America, San Francisco, CA.

Collins, C., Stommel, M., Thiele, J., Given, C. W., & King, S. (1989). *Knowledge and use of community services among family caregivers of Alzheimer's patients.* Unpublished manuscript.

Couper, D., & Sheehan, N. (1987). Family dynamics: An educational model for adult children caregivers. *Family Relations, 36,* 181–186.

Deimling, G. T., & Bass, D. M. (1986). Symptoms of mental impairment among elderly adults and their effects on family caregivers. *Journal of Gerontology, 41,* 778–784.

Fiore, J., Coppel, D. B., Becker, J., & Cox, G. B. (1986). Social support as a multi-faceted concept: Examination of important dimensions for adjustment. *American Journal of Community Psychology, 14,* 93–111.

Fitting, M., Rabins, P., Lucas, M. J., & Eastham, J. (1986). Caregivers for dementia patients: A comparison of husbands and wives. *The Gerontologist, 26,* 248–252.

Frankfather, D., Smith, M. J., & Caro, F. (1981). *Family care of the elderly: Public initiatives & private obligations.* Lexington, MA: Lexington Books.

Gallagher, D. (1985). Intervention strategies to assist caregivers of frail elders: Current research status and future research directions. In M. P. Lawton & G. Maddox (Eds.), *Annual Review of Gerontology and Geriatrics, 5* (pp. 249–282). New York: Springer Publishing Co.

Gilhooly, M. (1984). The impact of caregiving on care-givers: Factors associated with the psychological well-being of people supporting a dementing relative in the community. *British Journal of Medical Psychology, 57,* 35–44.

Given, B., & Given, C. W. (1989). *Family home care for cancer: A community-based model* (Grant #1 R01 NR01915). Rockville, MD: National Center for Nursing Research.

Given, B., King, S., Collins, C., & Given, C. W. (1988, October). Family caregivers of the elderly: Involvement and reactions to care. *Archives of Psychiatric Nursing, II,* 281–288.

Given, C. W., Collins, C. E., & Given, B. A. (1988). Sources of stress among families caring for relatives with Alzheimer's disease. *Nursing Clinics of North America, 23*(1), 69–82.

Given, C. W., & Given, B. (1988a). *Caregiver responses to managing elderly patients at home* (Grant #1 R01 AG06584). Rockville, MD: DHHS National Institute on Aging. Year II Progress Report.

Given, C. W., & Given, B. (1988b). *Impact of Alzheimer's Disease on family caregivers* (Grant #1 R01 MH41766). Rockville, MD: DHHS National Institute of Mental Health.

Given, C. W., & Given, B. (1989). *Caregiver responses to managing elderly patients at home* (Grant #2 R01 AG06584). Rockville, MD: DHHS National Institute on Aging. Principal Investigator, Charles W. Given.

Given, C. W., Given, B., & Ogle, K. (1988, November). *Measurement of intensity of involvement of family in caring for patients at home.* Paper presented at the 41st

Annual Scientific Meeting of the Gerontological Society of America, San Francisco, CA.

Given, C. W., Stommel, M., Zemach, R., Given B., Collins, C., King, S., & Vredevoogd, J. (1988). *Conceptualization and measurement of family members' involvement in caregiving.* Unpublished manuscript.

Gwyther, L. P., & George, L. K. (1986). Caregivers for dementia patients: Complex determinants of well-being and burden. *The Gerontologist, 26,* 245–247.

Haley, W. E., Levine, E. G., Brown, S. L., & Bartolucci, A. A. (1987). Stress, appraisal, coping, and social support as predictors of adaptational outcome among dementia caregivers. *Psychology and Aging, 2,* 323–330.

Haley, W. E., & Pardo, K. M. (1989). Relationship of severity of dementia to caregiving stressors. *Psychology and Aging, 4,* 389–392.

Hirshfield, M. (1983). Homecare vs. institutionalization: Family caregiving and senile brain disease. *International Journal of Nursing Studies, 20,* 23–32.

Horowitz, A. (1985a). Family caregiving to the frail elderly. In C. Eisdorfer (Ed.), *Annual Review of Gerontology & Geriatrics, 5,* (pp. 194–246). New York: Springer Publishing Co.

Horowitz, A. (1985b). Sons and daughters as caregivers to older parents: Differences in role performance and consequences. *The Gerontologist, 25,* 612–617.

Johnson, C. L. (1983). Dyadic family relations and social support. *The Gerontologist, 23,* 377–383.

Kahan, J., Kemp, B., Staples, F. R., & Brummel-Smith, K. (1985). Decreasing the burden in families caring for relative with a dementing illness: A controlled study. *Journal of American Geriatric Society, 33,* 665–670.

Kiecolt-Glaser, J. K., Glaser, R., Shuttleworth, E. C., Dyer, C. S., Orocki, P., & Speicher, C. E. (1987). Chronic stress and immunity in family caregivers of Alzheimer's disease victims. *Psychosomatic Medicine, 49,* 523–35.

Kiecolt-Glaser, J. K., & Glaser, R. (1989). Caregiving, mental health, and immune function. In E. Light & B. D. Lebowitz, (Eds.), *Alzheimer's disease treatment and family stress: Directions for research.* Rockville, MD: U.S. Department of Health and Human Services.

Kosberg, J. I., & Cairl, R. E. (1986). The cost of care index: A case management tool for screening informal care providers. *The Gerontologist, 26,* 273–278.

Krause, N. (1987). Understanding the stress process: Linking social support with locus of control. *Journal of Gerontology, 42,* 589–593.

Kuypers, J. A., & Bengston, V. L. (1983). Toward competence in the older family. In T. Brubaker (Ed.), *Family relationships in later life* (pp. 211–238). Beverly Hills, CA: Sage.

Lang, A. M., & Brody, E. M. (1983). Characteristics of middle-aged daughters and help to their elderly mothers. *Journal of Marriage and the Family, 45,* 193–202.

Lawton, M. P., Brody, E. M., & Saperstein, A. R. (1989). A controlled study of respite service for caregivers of Alzheimer's patients. *The Gerontologist, 29,* 8–16.

Lawton, M. P., Kleban, M. H., Moss, M., Rovine, M., & Glicksman, A. (1989). Measuring caregiving appraisal. *Journal of Gerontology, 44,* 61–71.

Lyles, J., King, S., & Given, B. (1990). *Social interaction, instrumental support and family caregiver perception of support.* Unpublished manuscript.

Mace, N. (1986). Caregiving aspects of Alzheimer's disease. *Business and Health, 3,* 32–38.

Manton, K. G. (1990). Epidemiological, demographic, and social correlates of disability among the elderly. *The Milbank Quarterly, 67*(Suppl), 13–58.

McCorkle, R., Benoliel, J., Donaldson, G., Georgiadou, F., Moinpour, C. & Goodell, B. (1989). A randomized clinical trial of home nursing care for lung cancer patients. *Cancer, 64,* 1375–1382.

Miller, B. (1987). Gender and control among spouses of the cognitively impaired: A research note. *The Gerontologist, 27,* 447–453.

Mohide, E. A., Torrance, G. W., Streiner, D. L., Pringle, D. M., & Gilbert, R. (1988). Measuring the well-being of family caregivers using the time trade-off technique. *Journal of Clinical Epidemiology, 41,* 475–482.

Montgomery, R. J. V. (1989). Investigating caregiver burden. In K. Markides & C. Cooper (Eds.), *Aging, stress, and health* (pp, 201–218). New York: Wiley.

Montgomery, R. J. V., Gonyea, J. G., & Hooyman, N. R. (1985). Caregiving and the experience of subjective and objective burden. *Family Relations, 34,* 19–26.

Moritz, D. J., Kasl, S. V., & Berkman, L. F. (1989). The health impact of living with a cognitively impaired elderly spouse: Depressive symptoms and social functioning. *Journal of Gerontology, 44,* 517–527.

Motenko, A. K. (1989). The frustrations, gratifications, and well-being of dementia caregivers. *The Gerontologist, 29,* 166–172.

National Long Term Care Channelling Demonstration. (1986). *Informal care to the impaired elderly: Report of the National Long Term Care Demonstration Survey of Informal Caregivers.* Contract # 100-80-0157. Plainsboro, NJ: U.S. Department of Health and Human Services Mathematics Policy Research Inc.

Noelker, L. S., & Bass, D. M. (1989). Home care for elderly persons: Linkages between formal and informal caregiving. *Journal of Gerontology: Social Sciences, 44,* 563–570.

Noelker, L. S., & Poulshock, S. W. (1982). *The effects on families of caring for impaired elderly in residence.* Washington, DC: Final Report Submitted to the Administration on Aging.

Noelker, L. S., & Wallace, R. W. (1985). The organization of family care for impaired elderly. *Journal of Family Issues, 6,* 23–44.

Oberst, M. T. (1989). *Family caregiving: Appraisal, coping, and outcomes.* Unpublished manuscript.

Oberst, M. J., & James, R. H. (1985). Going home: Patient and spouse adjustment following cancer surgery. *Topics in Clinical Nursing, 7*(1), 46–57.

Oberst, M. T., & Scott, D. W. (1988). Post discharge distress in surgically treated cancer patients and their spouses. *Research in Nursing and Health, 11,* 223–233.

Office of Technology Assessment. (1987). *Losing a million minds: Confronting the tragedy of Alzheimer's Disease and other dementias* (OTA BA 323). Washington, DC: U.S. Government Printing Office.

Pagel, M., Becker, J., & Coppel, D. (1985). Loss of control, self-blame and depression: An investigation of spouse caretakers of Alzheimer's Disease patients. *Journal of Abnormal Psychology, 94,* 169–182.

Pearson, J., Verma, S., & Nellett, C. (1988). Elderly psychiatric patient status and caregiver perceptions as predictors of caregiver burden. *The Gerontologist, 28,* 79–83.

Phillips, L. R. (1983). Abuse/neglect of the frail elderly at home: An exploration of theoretical relationship. *Journal of Advanced Nursing, 8,* 379–392.

Phillips, L. R., & Rempusheski, V. F. (1985). A decision making model for diagnosing and intervening in elder abuse and neglect. *Nursing Research, 34*, 134–139.

Phillips, L. R., & Rempusheski, V. F. (1986). Caring for the frail elderly at home: Toward a theoretical explanation of the dynamics of poor quality family caregiving. *Advances in Nursing Science, 8*(4), 62–84.

Pinkston, E. M., & Linsk, N. L. (1984). Behavioral family intervention with the impaired elderly. *The Gerontologist, 24*, 576–583.

Poulshock, S. W., & Deimling, G. T. (1984). Families caring for elders in residence: Issues in the measurement of burden. *Journal of Gerontology, 39*, 230–239.

Pratt, C. C., Schmall, V. L., Wright, S., & Cleland, M. (1985). Burden and coping strategies of caregivers to Alzheimer's patients. *Family Relations, 34*, 27–33.

Priddy, J., & Gallagher, D. (1985). *Clinical and research issues in the study of caregiver support groups.* Baltimore, MD: National Institute on Aging.

Pruchno, R., & Resch, N. (1989). Husbands and wives as caregivers: Antecedents of depression and burden. *The Gerontologist, 29*, 159–165.

Quayhagen, M. P., & Quayhagen, M. (1988). Alzheimer's stress: Coping with the caregiving role. *The Gerontologist, 28*, 391–396.

Quayhagen, M. P., & Quayhagen, M. (1989). Differential effects of family-based strategies on Alzheimer's disease. *The Gerontologist, 29*, 150–155.

Rabins, P. V., Mace, N. L., & Lucas, M. J. (1982). The impact of dementia on the family. *Journal of the American Medical Association, 248*, 333–335.

Reece, D., Walz, T., & Hageboeck, H. (1983). Intergenerational care providers of non-institutionalized frail elderly: Characteristics and consequences. *Journal of Gerontological Social Work, 5*, 21–34.

Rempusheski, V. F. , & Phillips, L. R. (1988). Elder versus caregivers: Games they play. *Geriatric Nursing, 9*, 30–34.

Robinson, B. (1983). Validation of a caregiver strain index. *The Journal of Gerontology, 38*, 344–348.

Robinson, B., & Thurnher, M. (1979). Taking care of aged parents: A family cycle transition. *The Gerontologist, 19*, 586–592.

Robinson, K. M. (1988). A social skills training program for adult caregivers. *Advances in Nursing Science, 10*(2), 59–72.

Romeis, J. C. (1989). Caregiver strain: Toward an enlarged perspective. *Journal of Aging & Health, 1*, 188–208.

Sager, A. (1983). A proposal for promoting more adequate long-term care for the elderly. *The Gerontologist, 23*, 13–17.

Satariano, W. A., Minkler, M. A., & Langhauser, C. (1984). The significance of an ill spouse for assessing health differences in an elderly population. *Journal of the American Geriatrics Society, 32*, 187–190.

Schulz, R., Biegel, D., Morycz, R., & Visintainer, P. (1989). Psychological paradigms for understanding caregiving. In E. Light & B. Lebowitz (Eds.), *Alzheimer's Disease treatment and family stress: Directions for research* (pp. 106–121). Rockville, MD: U.S. Dept of Health and Human Services.

Schulz, R., Tompkins, C., & Rau, M. (1990). A longitudinal study of the psychosocial impact of stroke on primary support persons. *Psychology and Aging, 3*, 131–141.

Scott, J. P., Roberto, K. A., & Hutton, T. H. (1986). Families of Alzheimer's victims: Family support to the caregivers. *Journal of the American Geriatrics Society, 34*, 348–354.

Shapiro, E., & Tuti, R. (1988). Who is really at risk of institutionalization? *The Gerontologist, 28,* 237–245.

Sheehan, N. W., & Nuttall, P. (1988). Conflict, emotion, and personal strain among family caregivers. *Family Relations, 37*(1), 92–98.

Silliman, R. A., & Sternberg, J. (1988). Family caregiving: Impact of patient functioning and underlying causes of dependency. *The Gerontologist, 28,* 377–382.

Silverstone, B., & Hyman, H. K. (1982). *You and your aging parents.* New York: Pantheon Books.

Smallegan, M. (1985). There was nothing else to do: Needs for care before nursing home admission. *The Gerontologist, 25,* 364–369.

Soldo, B. J., & Myllyluoma, J. (1983). Caregivers who live with dependent elderly. *The Gerontologist, 23,* 605–611.

Springer, D., & Brubaker, T. H. (1984). *Family caregivers and dependent elderly: Minimizing stress and maximizing independence.* Beverly Hills, CA: Sage.

Stetz, K. M. (1987). Caregiving demands during advanced cancer. *Cancer Nursing, 10,* 260–268.

Stetz, K. M., & Hanson, W. K. (1989). *Caregiving demands during advanced cancer: Alterations in perception during and after the experience.* Unpublished manuscript.

Stetz, K. M., & Johnson, R. W. (1989). The relationship among background characteristics, purpose in life, and caregiving demands on health of spouse caregivers. *Scholarly Inquiry for Nursing Practice: An International Journal, 3,* 133–153.

Stoller, E. P., & Earl, L. L. (1983). Help with activities of everyday life: Sources of support for the noninstitutionalized elderly. *The Gerontologist, 23,* 64–70.

Stoller, E. P., & Pugliesi, K. L. (1989). Other roles of caregivers: Competing responsibilities or supportive resources. *Journal of Gerontology, 44,* 231–238.

Stommel, M., Given, C. W., & Given, B. (1990). Depression as an overriding variable explaining caregiver burdens. *Journal of Aging and Health, 2,* 81–102.

Stone, R., Cafferata, G. L., & Sangle, J. (1987). Caregivers of the frail elderly: A national profile. *The Gerontologist, 27,* 616–626.

Tennestedt, S. L., McKinley, J. B., & Sullivan, L. M. (1989). Informal care for frail elders: The role of secondary caregivers. *The Gerontologist, 29,* 677–683.

Teri, L., Borson, S., Kiyak, A., & Yamagishi, M. (1989). Behavioral disturbance, cognitive dysfunction, and functional skill: Prevalence and relationship in Alzheimer's disease. *Journal of the American Geriatrics Society, 37,* 109–116.

Treas, J., Gronvold, R., & Bengston, V. L. (1980). *Filial destiny? The effect of birth order on relations with aging parents.* Paper presented at the Annual Scientific Meeting of the Gerontological Society of America, San Diego, CA.

Vess, J., Moreland, J., & Schwebel, A. I. (1985). Understanding family role reallocation following a death: A theoretical framework. *Omega, 16,* 115–128.

Vitaliano, P. P. (1988). *Correlates of mental health in DAT spouses* (Grant #1 RO1 MH43267-01). Rockville, MD: National Institute of Mental Health.

Weissert, W. G., Cready, C. M., & Pawelak, J. E. (1988). The past and future of home and community-based long-term care. *The Milbank Quarterly, 66,* 309–338.

Wellisch, D., Landsverk, J., Guidera, K., Pasnau, R., & Fawzy, F. (1983). Evaluation of psychosocial problems of the homebound cancer patient: Methodology and problem frequencies. *Psychosomatic Medicine, 45,* 11–21.

Wilson, H. S. (1989a). Family caregiving for a relative with Alzheimer's dementia: Coping with negative choices. *Nursing Research, 38,* 94–98.

Wilson, H. S. (1989b). Family caregivers: The experience of Alzheimer's disease. *Applied Nursing Research, 2,* 40–45.

Worcester, M. I., & Quayhagen, M. P. (1983). Correlates of caregiving satisfaction: Prerequisites to elder home care. *Research in Nursing and Health, 6,* 61–67.

Yankelovich, Skelley, & White, Inc. (1986). *Caregivers of patients with dementia.* Washington, DC: Office of Technology Assessment, U.S. Congress. U.S. Government Printing Office.

Young, R., & Kahana, E. (1989). Specifying caregiver outcomes: Gender and relationship aspects of caregiving strain. *The Gerontologist, 29,* 660–666.

Zarit, S. H. (1989). Issues and directions in family intervention research. In E. Light, & B. D. Lebowitz (Eds.), *Alzheimer's disease treatment and family stress: Directions for research* (pp. 458–486). DHHS publication #ADM 89-1569. Rockville, MD: U.S. Department of Health and Human Services.

Zarit, S. H., Reever, K. E., & Bach-Peterson, J. (1980). Relatives of the impaired elderly: Correlates of feelings of burden. *The Gerontologist, 20,* 649–655.

Zarit, S. H., Todd, P. A., & Zarit, J. M. (1986). Subjective burden of husbands and wives as caregivers: A longitudinal study. *The Gerontologist, 26,* 260–266.

Zarit, S. H., & Zarit, J. M. (1982). Families under stress: Interventions for caregivers of senile dementia patients. *Psychotherapy, Theory, Research and Practice, 19,* 461–471.

CARL A. RUDISILL LIBRARY
LENOIR-RHYNE COLLEGE

Chapter 5

Family Adaptation to a Child's Chronic Illness

JOAN KESSNER AUSTIN

SCHOOL OF NURSING

INDIANA UNIVERSITY

CONTENTS

Overview of Selected Articles
Approaches
Assumptions
Design and Sampling
Instrument Development
Major Findings
Effect on Family Members
Effect on Mother–Infant Interactions
Family Adaptation Processes
*Relationships Between Family Characteristics
and Child Attributes*
Recommendations for Future Research

Approximately 10% to 15% of children under 18 years of age have a chronic physical illness or condition (Perrin, 1985). According to Gortmaker (1985), the number of children with chronic conditions has increased substantially in recent decades. Nursing is one of many disciplines that is actively investigating how family members adapt to a chronic health condition in a child. In this chapter research in the nursing literature related to family adaptation to a chronic illness or disability in a child is reviewed. Theoretical approaches,

This review was supported in part by a grant, NS22416, from the National Institute of Neurological Disorders and Stroke, United States Public Health Service. The author gratefully acknowledges the contributions of Carol Trout, R. N., M.S.N to the literature search and compiling of references.

103

underlying assumptions, and research methods utilized in the studies are described and critiqued. Major findings are summarized in four areas: effect on family members, effect on mother–infant interactions, family adaptation processes, and relationships between family characteristics and child attributes. Gaps in the literature are identified and recommendations are made for future research.

Various strategies were used to search the nursing literature from 1974 to 1989. Computer searches of the Cumulative Index to Nursing and Allied Health Literature and MEDLINE were used for family and chronic illness. Hand searches were performed for the current contents of nursing journals and the references from recently published articles. In addition, family nurse researchers active in the field were contacted for articles. Although this review was almost exclusively a review of the nursing literature, a few articles by nurse authors published in interdisciplinary journals also were included.

Published studies were included if they pertained to research on any aspect of family adaptation to chronic illness or disability in a child. Reports of studies were considered to be research if the sample was described, purposive data collection (i.e., to answer research questions or test hypotheses) occurred, and data were analyzed. Articles in which researchers used case studies to describe further the concepts used in the development of theory also were included.

Chronic illness or condition was defined as physical impairment that rarely is cured, is characterized by both acute episodes and stable periods, and interferes with the maximum functioning of the individual (Thomas, 1984). Even though the primary focus in this review was on chronic physical conditions that generally are not life threatening (e.g., epilepsy, diabetes, cerebral palsy, and congenital anomalies), studies with samples that included children with life-threatening conditions (e.g., cancer) were included in some studies with heterogeneous samples. Cystic fibrosis was included because it is generally chronic during childhood, with death usually not occurring until early adulthood.

The concepts of adaptation and family were defined broadly. Adaptation was defined as any response to the chronic illness by a family member. Articles were included if data had been collected from at least one family member, including siblings, and pertained to at least one family member's adaptation to the chronic illness in the child.

OVERVIEW OF SELECTED ARTICLES

Of the 39 research articles included in the final review, approximately one-third were published in nursing research journals and two-thirds in clinical journals. Authors focused on concept and theory development in 5 articles and reported results from completed research in 28 articles. An additional six articles on instruments developed also were selected for review.

Approaches

Both inductive and deductive research approaches were well represented. Researchers used the inductive approach primarily in qualitative studies, generally focusing on family perceptions and the processes used to cope with a chronic illness in a child (e.g., Anderson, 1981; Anderson & Chung, 1982; Deatrick, Knafl, & Walsh, 1988). Researchers whose studies used the deductive approach generally used quantitative methods and focused on the effect of the child with a chronic condition on other family members (e.g., Van Cleve, 1989) or on relationships between family characteristics and child attributes (e.g., Khampalikit, 1983). Only a few researchers (e.g., Austin, McBride, & Davis, 1984) used a combination of approaches and methods as suggested by Knafl and Deatrick (1987) and Moriarity (1990).

In approximately one-half of the studies researchers included theoretical frameworks for the research, with the majority using a stress framework. Seven studies by researchers Austin (Austin, 1988; Austin, McBride, & Davis, 1984; Austin & McDermott, 1988) and McCubbin (McCubbin, 1984; 1988, 1989; McCubbin & Huang, 1989) were based on the Double ABCX Model of Family Adaptation to Stress (McCubbin & Patterson, 1983). Four other studies by Cappuzzi (1980), Gibson (1986), Schlomann (1988) and Van Cleve (1989) were based on stress frameworks, such as Lazarus' theory of stress and coping (Lazarus, 1966) and crisis theory (e.g., Moos & Tsu, 1977). Attachment theory (Bowlby, 1969) was used by Capuzzi (1989), Holaday (1981), and Mercer (1974), and systems theory (Johnson, 1980) was used by Holaday (1982; 1987) and Van Cleve (1989). Social learning theory (Bandura, 1972) and self-care theory (Orem, 1971) were used, respectively, by King (1981) and by Kruger, Shawver, and Jones (1980). The theories selected by nurse scientists are similar to those used by family scientists in other disciplines (S. Murphy, 1986).

Assumptions

Assumptions made about the nature of the family's response to having a child with a chronic condition varied. The most common assumption was that the onset of a chronic condition in a child is a stressful event for the entire family. Some researchers further assumed that chronic illness is a continuing source of stress that can result in more stress-related problems for the family with a child with a chronic illness than would be found in families whose children were healthy (Stullenbarger, Norris, Edgil, & Prosser, 1987). In this view, both the child with the chronic condition and the family members were considered potential victims of the chronic condition. These researchers generally studied the effect of the condition on the family members (e.g., Horner, Rawlins, & Giles, 1987) or on the interactions between family members and the chronically ill child (e.g., King, 1981). Other researchers made no assumptions about the nature of the interaction between the child with the chronic condition and the family, and, subsequently, focused on the family members' subjective meanings in relation to the chronic condition and the processes families used to deal with it (e.g., Anderson, 1981).

Still other researchers assumed a dynamic relationship between the chronically ill child and the family members. These researchers generally studied relationships between family characteristics and attributes of the child's adaptation (e.g., Austin, 1988) or health status (e.g., McCubbin, 1988), with the goal of identifying which family characteristics were linked with positive or negative outcomes in the child with the chronic illness.

There is some support in the literature for each of the foregoing assumptions, especially for the assumption that the onset of chronic illness in a child is stressful to the family. Findings from several studies indicate strong reciprocal effects between the ill child and the family, whereby the family both affects and is affected by the illness (Shapiro, 1983). There is less support, however, for the assumption that all families, regardless of severity of the chronic condition, are experiencing more stress than families from the general population (Trute & Hauch, 1988). The broader perspective, which allows for both positive and negative influences of a chronic condition in a child on the family (Burr, 1985), is the prevailing view based on recent research in other health care disciplines.

Design and Sampling

Approximately one-half of the studies reviewed were descriptive and about one-third were correlational. Almost one-fifth included a comparison sample. Only four researchers (Capuzzi, 1989; Holaday, 1981; 1982; 1987; Mercer, 1974; K. M. Murphy, 1990) used prospective, longitudinal designs. No studies were found that had an experimental or evaluation research design.

A review of the sampling strategies revealed two diverse views. One view was that chronic conditions are very similar in their effect on the family, and, consequently, vastly different conditions were grouped together when studying family adaptation. An opposing view was that chronic conditions vary greatly in characteristics (e.g., predictability, obviousness of impairment, level of incapacitation, prognosis, and cause) and either should be studied separately or controlled for in the design. Investigators subscribing to the latter view generally used samples that were homogeneous in regard to the chronic illness. In approximately one-half of the studies reviewed several chronic conditions were grouped together without an effort to compare and contrast differences in family responses to them. In a few of these studies both life-threatening and nonlife-threatening conditions were studied without taking characteristics of the illness or type of illness as an independent or intervening variable (e.g., Anderson, 1981). Both views regarding whether chronic illnesses should be studied as a group or studied individually have been supported in the literature outside of nursing (Pless & Perrin, 1985; Rolland, 1988).

Instrument Development

Two nurse researchers developed instruments that specifically measured aspects of family adaptation to a chronic condition in a child. Hymovich (1981; 1983; 1984) designed an instrument to measure parental perceptions of the impact of a chronic childhood condition both on the family and on the family's coping strategies. The most recent version of the instrument, Hymovich's Parent Perception Inventory (Hymovich, 1990), contained six separate scales: concerns, beliefs and feelings, coping, general information, siblings, and spouse concerns and coping. Internal consistency reliability (Cronbach's alpha) ranged from .33 to .90; stability reliability (r) ranged from .74 to .92 (Hymovich, 1990). More research is needed to determine the psychometric properties of the newest version of this self-report instrument.

The Coping Health Inventory for Parents (CHIP) is a 45-item self-report questionnaire developed by McCubbin and her colleagues (McCubbin, 1984; McCubbin et al., 1983) that measures parental coping with a chronic illness in a child. Using factor analysis, three coping patterns were identified: Maintaining Family Integration, Co-operation, and An Optimistic Definition of the Situation; Maintaining Social Support, Self-Esteem, and Psychological Stability; and Understanding the Health Care Situation Through Communication With Other Parents and Consultation With the Health Care Team. Internal consistency reliabilities (Cronbach's alpha) ranged from .71 to .79 (McCubbin, 1984).

MAJOR FINDINGS

Major findings from the research are grouped in four areas: effect on family members, effect on mother–infant interactions, family adaptation processes, and relationships between family characteristics and child attributes. The literature is described and critiqued in each area.

Effect on Family Members

General Effect. The effect of a chronic illness in a child on family members was described in seven studies, with researchers in four studies focusing primarily on parents (Hodges & Parker, 1987; Horner et al., 1987; McKeever, 1981; Waechter, 1977) and researchers in three focusing on siblings (Kruger et al., 1980; Pinyerd, 1983; Taylor, 1980). One study (Horner et al., 1987) was a survey of a rather large sample ($N = 164$). In the remaining studies researchers gathered data through semi-structured interviews with smaller convenience samples ($N = 10$ to $N = 50$). All studies were exploratory in nature. Five of the six studies were retrospective and involved one data collection. Although one study (Waechter, 1977) was described as a prospective design with one data collection at birth and follow-up interviews at 3-month intervals, findings over time were not addressed specifically. The reliability and validity of instruments generally were not addressed adequately. In four studies (Hodges & Parker, 1987; Kruger et al., 1980; Pinyerd, 1983; Taylor, 1980) data were examined using content analysis and descriptive statistics. Samples in three of the studies consisted of children with a single chronic disease (i.e., diabetes, cystic fibrosis, and myelomeningocele), and in the other four a wide variety of conditions were represented. Even though authors alluded to theoretical frameworks, none of the studies specifically included testing of a theory. The major strength of these descriptive studies was the resulting suggested directions for future research.

Results were similar for the descriptive studies and generally indicated that a chronic condition in a child had an effect on the whole family. Emotional responses including shock, fear, anger, and guilt were found initially in parents' responses to the diagnosis of the condition (Hodges & Parker, 1987; McKeever, 1981; Waechter, 1977). Increased anxiety and need for coping were reported for both parents (Hodges & Parker, 1987) and siblings (Kruger et al., 1980; Pinyerd, 1983; Taylor, 1980). These findings were interesting because siblings often were given incomplete information by parents to keep them from worrying (Taylor, 1980). A common theme was parents' need for additional help and support from professionals in managing the medical regime (Hodges & Parker, 1987; Horner et al., 1987; McKeever, 1981). Other problems identified for parents were dealing with the chronic condition at school (Hodges & Parker, 1987), financial strain (Horner et al., 1987), dealing with the unpredictability of the chronic condition and its effect on the child's future (McKeever, 1981; Waechter, 1977), and difficulty in talking with siblings about the condition (Taylor, 1980). Siblings reported that they felt isolated, had less time with their parents, had family-activity plans disrupted, and had their chores increased as a result of the illness in a brother or sister (Kruger et al., 1980; Pinyerd, 1983; Taylor, 1980).

Although the majority of the researchers reported only on negative effects on the family from the chronic condition, it should be noted that the effect on the marital relationship was positive in 5 of 10 fathers interviewed by McKeever (1981). In addition, Taylor (1980) found that one-third of the siblings derived some benefits from having a sister or brother with a chronic illness, including increased cooperation, self-esteem, empathy, and cognitive mastery.

Effect in Specific Areas.   In seven studies investigators focused on specific effects of the child with a chronic illness on the family and identified variables associated with these changes. Two were comparison studies (King, 1981; McCubbin, 1989) and five were correlational studies (Austin et al., 1984; Austin & McDermott, 1988; Gibson, 1986; Schlomann, 1988; Van Cleve, 1989). With the exception of King (1981), who used Bandura's Social Learning Theory (1972) as a framework, the rest were based on a stress theoretical framework. All researchers used instruments with adequate reliability and validity.

Very few differences were found in the comparison studies. McCubbin (1989) compared one- and two-parent families coping with a child with cerebral palsy on 14 dimensions of stress and strength. Contrary to expectations, single-parent families did not experience more stress than two-parent families. Differences were found in three of the areas, with single-parent families having more adaptability, fewer financial resources, and lower levels of coping related to family maintenance than two-parent families. A strength of this study was the matching of the two groups on severity of illness of the child as well as on the age and gender of the parent. The small samples ($n = 27$ for each group) and the wide age range of the children were limitations. Among parents who had both children with a chronic illness and healthy children, King (1981) found no differences for type of child in parenting behaviors of punishment, promotion of independence, rules of behavior, and amount of spouse involvement. The small sample ($n = 19$ parent dyads) and the wide diversity in type of chronic condition in the children were limitations.

In the two correlational studies by Austin and colleagues (Austin, McBride, & Davis, 1984; Austin & McDermott, 1988), positive relationships were found between parental attitudes toward epilepsy and aspects of parental adaptation in parents of school-aged children with epilepsy. Positive attitudes were linked with increased use of the coping behaviors of family maintenance and social support (Austin & McDermott, 1988) and higher levels of parental adjustment to epilepsy (Austin et al., 1984). An exploration of gender differences indicated that the relationships were significant only for mothers. The small number of fathers in the sample ($n = 17$) warranted cautious interpretation of gender differences. A hypothesized positive relationship between parents' beliefs and attitudes about their child's condition and parental coping strategies was not supported in the Von Cleve (1989) study of 100 parents of children with spina bifida. The lack of relationship between the attitude and coping measures may have resulted from the more general measurement of attitude in contrast to coping behavior. Van Cleve did find parental coping positively related to quality of the marital relationship, marital satisfaction, and attendance in a support group.

In a study of coping behaviors of 56 parents whose children had cystic fibrosis, Gibson (1986) found that parents reported social support and concentrating on positive aspects of the situation to be the most helpful coping strategies. Also, fathers directed less effort toward family maintenance than mothers. The small number of fathers ($n = 10$) rendered these results only suggestive. Schlomann (1988) studied the interrelationship among five areas of developmental delay and seven areas of impact on the family and found larger developmental gaps associated with greater negative effect on the family. The small sample ($N = 20$), the large number of correlations carried out, and the wide range in type of chronic condition (e.g., gastrointestinal disorder to Down's Syndrome) are limitations.

Effect on Mother–Infant Interactions

Three studies that focused on interactions between mothers and infants with handicaps were reported in five articles (Capuzzi, 1989; Holaday, 1981; 1982; 1987; Mercer, 1974). All three studies had prospective, longitudinal designs with structured observation data-collection methods. In addition, investigators reported adequate reliability of measures. Even though samples were small, the large number of observations and the attention to reliability and validity of the data enhanced credibility of the findings.

In a study of five mothers and their infants with handicaps, Mercer (1974) hypothesized that mothers' responses to their infants would be predominantly aversive in the first 2 months and change to predominantly attachment by 3 months. Contrary to expectations, maternal attachment responses predominated over aversion responses in the initial period. Two researchers, Capuzzi (1989) and Holaday (1981, 1982, 1987) compared mothers' interactions with infants with a chronic illness to those of mothers of healthy infants. Holaday conducted four observations each on 6 mother–infant dyads between 4 and 6 months postpartum. She observed that infants with a chronic illness cried more frequently than healthy infants regardless of the mother's responses to the cry (1981). Mothers of healthy infants were more apt to inattend selectively to some infant cries than mothers of infants with chronic illness who attended to almost every cry (Holaday, 1982). In five of the dyads of infants with handicaps, atypical patterns of interaction were found where mothers engaged in interruptive behavior (e.g., interrupting the infant when it was quiet). Holaday (1987) discussed the possibility that mothers of children with a handicap may be at risk for overstimulating their infants. When Capuzzi (1989) compared maternal–infant attachment behaviors of 15 mothers of infants with handicaps with 21 mothers of healthy infants, differences were found at 1 month postpartum but not at 6 and 12 months. No differences in maternal attachment behaviors were found, however, when the effects of the mother's prenatal social support were partialed out, indicating that social support buffers the effect of the infant's handicap on maternal attachment behaviors. The use of multiple regression with such a small sample, however, can lead to unstable and inconsistent results (Prescott, 1987).

Family Adaptation Processes

Family adaptation processes were the focus of 9 articles in which 5 of the researchers (Anderson, 1981; Anderson & Chung, 1982; Deatrick, Knafl, & Walsh, 1988; Knafl & Deatrick, 1986; Krulik, 1980) investigated the normalization process. Researchers in an additional four studies (Deatrick & Knafl, 1990; Gallo, 1990; Knafl & Deatrick, 1990; K. M. Murphy, 1990) focused on family management styles. All researchers employed inductive approaches and qualitative methods. A strength of these studies was the authors building on previous findings in the development of their own research. A limitation of these studies was the small amount of information reported on the specifics of the qualitative methods, which made it difficult to evaluate the validity of the analyses. Examples and case studies provided rich descriptive data, however, to support conclusions.

The first study in the nursing literature that included a description of normalization behaviors of parents of chronically ill children was by Krulik (1980). She described successful normalization tactics used by 20 mothers to minimize their children's feelings of being different. Krulik studied children with life-threatening conditions as well as children with chronic illness. In general, normalization strategies enhanced the child's coping behaviors and resources and modified the environment to better accommodate the child.

In two studies that were focused primarily on normalization behaviors of families, Anderson (1981) compared 4 families with children with a chronic illness who identified themselves as coping well with 12 families with healthy children. She identified an inconsistency in the use of normalization; parents deemphasized the deviance of the child with the chronic illness while family members were making many adjustments in the family lifestyle and changing expectations for the child. Consequently, the child with the illness was given the conflicting message of "you are normal" and "you are different." A major conclusion in the second study (Anderson & Chung, 1982) was that the concept of normalization is culturally based. In a comparison of seven white families and six Chinese families with children with a chronic illness, normalization was a goal only of the white families. In contrast, the Chinese families' goal was to keep the chronically ill child content and happy.

In a 1986 study Knafl and Deatrick traced the origin and subsequent development of the concept of normalization. They concluded that four criteria needed to be met for normalization: (a) acknowledgment of the impairment in the child, (b) definition of the family life as essentially normal, (c) perceptions that the social consequences as a result of the illness were minimal, and (d) engagement in behaviors that communicated the normalcy of the child and the family to others. Using three case studies, the authors further differentiated normalization from the related but distinct concepts of denial and disassociation coping behaviors. In a 1988 study, Deatrick and associates found evidence of normalization in 11 of 12 families of children with osteogenesis imperfecta. For those 11 families the focus of the normalization behaviors was similar to that found by Krulik (1980): strengthening the child's coping resources and making the child's environment more accommodating to the special needs of the child.

In recent work Knafl and Deatrick (1990, p. 8) used concept analysis to develop an emerging conceptual model of family-management style with three interactive components: "definition of the situation, management behaviors, and sociocultural context." Two cases were used representing the two family management styles of normalization and conflictual. The family-management style framework was illustrated further using an indepth case study on juvenile diabetes by Gallo (1990). In addition, K. M. Murphy (1990) used the family-management style framework to study 20 mothers' and 20 fathers' responses to the birth of a high-risk infant over a 5-month period. Three dyadic management styles were found: agreement on socially prescribed management styles, adoption of parallel styles, and negotiation of a mutually interdependent style.

In further development of the family-management style framework, Deatrick and Knafl (1990) have conducted conceptual analysis of the family-management behaviors component. Family-management behaviors are behavioral accommodations made in response to the special needs of the child with the chronic illness. The authors propose that family members select behaviors to manage changes brought about by the child's illness on a day-to-day basis. These behaviors, which are based on each family member's perceptions of the total situation, can be understood by examining the goals, underlying conceptual dimensions, foci (i.e., child's illness, family system, and social system), and implementors of the behaviors.

Relationships Between Family Characteristics and Child Attributes

In five studies researchers investigated the relationships between family characteristics and child attributes (Austin, 1988; Khampalikit, 1983; McCubbin, 1988; McCubbin & Huang, 1989; Stullenbarger et al., 1987). All researchers utilized self-report questionnaires with adequate reliability and validity. All of the samples were homogeneous in regard to type of chronic illness studied, and two researchers (Austin, 1988; Khampalikit, 1983) used comparison groups to answer selected research questions. In addition, three researchers (Austin, 1988; Khampalikit, 1983; Stullenbarger et al., 1987) selected samples that were homogeneous in regard to developmental stage of the child. Samples were limited further to families of children who had had their respective conditions for a certain period of time in two studies (Austin, 1988; Stullenbarger et al., 1987).

In a study of 57 asthmatic and 47 healthy children, Khampalikit (1983) found that children with asthma were more dependent than the comparison group. The author found a positive low correlation ($r = -.27$ to .37) between mothers' perceptions of their children's asthma and their children's dependency. Stullenbarger et al. (1987) found no relationship between actual parenting style and competence behaviors in 26 children with cystic fibrosis; only ideal parenting style was a significant predictor of child competency. A major limitation of the study was the small sample for the use of multiple regression.

Austin (1988) examined the differences in family resources, family adaptation, and child adaptation between 54 children with epilepsy and 57 children with asthma. Children with epilepsy had significantly lower self-concepts and more behavior problems than children with asthma. In addition, families of children with epilepsy were found to have lower levels of adaptation and resources (i.e., esteem and communication, extended family social support, and financial well-being) than families of children with asthma. In a second portion of the study, children with poor adaptation to epilepsy (i.e., behavior problems and depression) were compared with children with good adaptation to epilepsy in regard to family resources and adaptation. Family resources and adaptation were significantly lower for children in the poor adaptation groups than for children in the good adaptation groups. Although children in the poor adaptation groups had significantly more seizures, seizure frequency was not controlled statistically in comparing of the two groups.

In two studies McCubbin (1988) and McCubbin and Huang (1989) investigated the amount of variance in the health status of children explained by family stress, resources, coping patterns, and family type. Strengths of these two studies were the inclusion of severity of illness as an independent variable in the design and the collection of data from both mothers and fathers. McCubbin (1988) studied 58 two-parent families of children with myelomeningocele. Relationships between family characteristics and child health were investigated using stepwise multiple regression in three sub-samples based on the severity of the myelomeningocele. More relationships were found between family characteristics and child health status in the severe group than in the mild and moderate groups. Thus, family system variables contributed more to the health status of the child when the child had more impairment. In addition, poor health in the child exacerbated the stress on the family and subsequently the response from the family.

McCubbin and Huang (1989) studied 130 two-parent families of children with cerebral palsy. Relationships between family characteristics (stress, types, resources, and parental coping) and child health (overall physical health and overall health improvement) were investigated using stepwise multiple regression in three subsamples based on severity of condition (i.e., mild, moderate, and severe). Again, differences in relationships between family characteristics were based on the severity of the condition. In the mildly impaired group, mother's coping strategies and family type contributed significantly to the overall improvement of the child's health status. In the moderately impaired group, family stress and family type contributed significantly to the child's overall physical health. In the severely impaired group three family characteristics—the resource of esteem/communication, mother's coping, and family type—contributed significantly to the overall improvement of the child's health status. No consistency was found in the family characteristics that had significant relationships with health status among the three groups. Even though findings in both of these studies should be interpreted with caution because of the small samples (Prescott, 1987) and the use of stepwise multiple regression (Aaronson, 1989), results suggested that severity of the illness may be a moderating variable that affects relationships between family characteristics and child attributes.

RECOMMENDATIONS FOR FUTURE RESEARCH

The ultimate goal of nursing care for families of children with a chronic illness is to facilitate adaptation to the condition that results in optimal physical and mental health of the child with the chronic illness and of the family. Current research in nursing does not provide a consistent body of knowledge about family adaptation to chronic illness in a child that would guide nursing practice. By far the majority of the research in the area is descriptive and is focused on individual parent responses to the child's chronic illness. Findings support strongly the proposition that chronic illness in a child may lead to stress for all family members. More information is needed, however, about the nature of the stress and the variables that affect stress. The findings that chronic illness can have positive effects on the marital relationship and on siblings suggest that researchers should determine factors that lead to positive effects on members of the family as well as on the child with the chronic illness. Potential positive effects in families when a child has a chronic illness need to be considered in the design of studies because the research approach taken affects the results found (Knafl & Deatrick, 1987). In addition, researchers have found that social support potentially buffers the effect of the chronic condition on maternal attachment behaviors. Therefore, future research should include designs that allow investigation of mediating variables.

Several trends in this body of research were similar to those noted by Feetham (1984) in a review of family research. First, researchers paid more attention to internal dynamics of the family rather than to the relationship between the family and external social structures. Second, even though family theories were used to frame the studies, many authors failed to develop the concept of family in the variables studied. According to Feetham (1984) these studies would be classified as family-related research. A third similar trend was that most researchers used the individual rather than the family as the unit of analysis. Although the use of only one family member as an informant can be criticized for not presenting a whole family view, collecting data from one family member may be preferable depending on the theory underlying the study and the purpose of the study (Thomas, 1987; Uphold & Strickland, 1989). In contrast to the trend found by Feetham (1984), the mother was not the primary source of information in these studies; data were collected from more than one family member in over one-half of the studies. In future research the strengths and limitations of the various ways to derive family scores from individual member's scores will need to be addressed (Thomas, 1987; Uphold & Strickland, 1989).

The stage-of-adaptation view, which is the most prevalent approach to conceptualizing family response to chronic illness in a child according to Shapiro (1983), rarely is mentioned and generally has not been taken into account in research designs. Excluding the longitudinal studies, time since onset of illness has not been a major variable. Parents going through various phases, such as denial and anger before reaching adaptation, are mentioned directly only by one author (Waechter, 1977). It may be that as families adapt to the chronic condition, more positive effects on the family are found or different family-management styles are employed. Research is needed to determine whether stages in family adaptation to chronic illness in a child affect family coping. Minimally, time-since-diagnosis should be considered in the design of a study. Longitudinal studies are needed to describe the natural history of the effect of the chronic condition both on the child and the family. For nursing practice, research is needed that describes family responses over time and that identifies factors leading to the best adaptive outcomes for the child and the family.

Representation of both inductive and deductive approaches strengthened this body of research. These diverse approaches with their associated different methods provide complementary perspectives on family adaptation to chronic illness. Future research could be enhanced through combinations of approaches and methods used in a given study. It was disappointing that researchers using the different approaches did not appear to be building on each other's work. For example, no deductive research to determine whether family normalization behaviors lead to successful child and family adaptation has been reported. Research is needed especially to follow up on Anderson's (1981) suggestion that normalization could have a negative effect on the child when a double message is given about being different. Knowledge about the relationship between family normalization behaviors and their effect on child adaptation to the chronic illness would provide a valuable basis for intervention studies.

The study of family adaptation to a chronic condition in a child is difficult because many variables potentially affect adaptation, including condition variables (e.g., age of onset, level of severity, prognosis, predictability of the symptoms, nature of limitations, and effect of treatment), demographic variables (e.g., socioeconomic status, size of family, culture), and child variables (e.g., age, gender, developmental stage, and ability to comprehend effect of the condition). Large samples are needed to accommodate more of these variables. One possibility is to select children with different illnesses but similar characteristics using a schema such as Rolland's (1987), in which illnesses are categorized according to psychosocial demands rather than by biological criteria.

McCubbins' (1988) finding that differences are based on severity of illness suggests that it is an important variable in the study of family adaptation to chronic illness and should be considered in the research design. Objective and subjective indicators of severity of illness may result in different findings. For example, Austin and colleagues (1984) report that parental perception of seizure control is a stronger predictor of parental adjustment than actual seizure frequency. Identification of relationships among disease characteristics, family characteristics, and child adaptation are critical if children and families at risk for adaptation problems are to be identified.

Developmental theory indicates that families have different tasks across the life span, and these normative tasks need to be considered in designing research on adaptation to chronic illness in a child. Research is needed to describe child and family adaptation at different developmental stages across the life cycle.

Excepting the studies of infants the large age range of the children with the chronic illness was a major weakness. Some authors failed to describe age or other characteristics of the children, whereas others included samples that spanned developmental levels from infancy to adulthood. Obtaining large samples of children who have the same or similar conditions or who are in the same developmental stage may be difficult, and authors reporting studies of diverse families should address the associated limitations.

Studies that test interventions aimed at enhancing family adaptation are greatly needed. Even though descriptive research supports that chronic childhood illness is stressful for families, no investigations of the effectiveness of educational or psychosocial interventions have been reported. Furthermore, level of psychosocial care was not considered a variable in any of the studies. Research that determines the nursing interventions leading to optimal outcomes for both the chronically ill child and the family will provide the needed foundation for nursing practice.

REFERENCES

Aaronson, L. S. (1989). A cautionary note on the use of stepwise regression. *Nursing Research, 38,* 309–311.

Anderson, J. M. (1981). The social construction of illness experience: Families with a chronically-ill child. *Journal of Advanced Nursing, 6,* 427–434.

Anderson, J., & Chung, J. (1982). Culture and illness: Parents' perceptions of their child's long term illness. *Nursing Papers/Perspectives in Nursing, 14*(4), 40–52.

Austin, J. K. (1988). Childhood epilepsy: Child adaptation and family resources. *Journal of Child and Adolescent Psychiatric and Mental Health Nursing, 1,* 18–24.

Austin, J. K., McBride, A. B., & Davis, H. W. (1984). Parental attitude and adjustment to childhood epilepsy. *Nursing Research, 33,* 92–96.

Austin, J. K., & McDermott, N. (1988). Parental attitude and coping behaviors of children with epilepsy. *Journal of Neuroscience Nursing, 20,* 174–179.

Bandura, A. (1972). *Social learning theory.* Englewood Cliffs, NJ: Prentice Hall.

Bowlby, J. (1969). *Attachment.* New York: Basic Books.

Burr, C. K. (1985). Impact on the family of a chronically ill child. In N. Hobbs & J. M. Perrin (Eds.), *Issues in the care of children with chronic illness* (pp. 24–40). San Francisco: Jossey-Bass.

Capuzzi, C. (1989). Maternal attachment to handicapped infants and the relationship to social support. *Research in Nursing & Health, 12,* 161–167.

Deatrick, J. A., & Knafl, K. A. (1990). Management behaviors: Day-to-day adjust-
ments in childhood chronic conditions. *Journal of Pediatric Nursing, 5,* 15–22.
Deatrick, J. A., Knafl, K. A., & Walsh, M. (1988). The process of parenting a child
with a disability: Normalization through accommodation. *Journal of Advanced
Nursing, 13,* 15–21.
Feetham, S. L. (1984). Family research: Issues and directions for nursing. In H. H.
Werley & J. F. Fitzpatrick (Eds.), *Annual Review of Nursing Research,* (pp.
3–25). New York: Springer Publishing Co.
Gallo, A. M. (1990). Family management style in juvenile diabetes: A case illustra-
tion. *Journal of Pediatric Nursing, 5,* 23–32.
Gibson, C. H. (1986). How parents cope with a child with cystic fibrosis. *Nursing
Papers/Perspectives in Nursing, 18*(3), 31–45.
Gortmaker, S. L. (1985). Demography of chronic childhood diseases. In N. Hobbs &
J. M. Perrin (Eds.), *Issues in the care of children with chronic illness* (pp.
135–154). San Francisco: Jossey-Bass.
Hodges, L. C., & Parker, J. (1987). Concerns of parents with diabetic children.
Pediatric Nursing, 13, 22–24, 68.
Holaday, B. (1981). Maternal responses to their chronically ill infants' attachment
behavior of crying. *Nursing Research, 30,* 343–348.
Holaday, B. (1982). Maternal conceptual set development: Identifying patterns of
maternal response to chronically ill infant crying. *Maternal Child Nursing
Journal, 11,* 47–59.
Holaday, B. (1987). Patterns of interaction between mothers and their chronically ill
children. *Maternal Child Nursing Journal, 16,* 29–45.
Horner, M. M., Rawlins, P., & Giles, K. (1987). How parents of children with
chronic conditions perceive their own needs. *The American Journal of Maternal
Child Nursing (MCN), 12,* 40–43.
Hymovich, D. P. (1981). Assessing the impact of chronic childhood illness on the
family and parent coping. *IMAGE: Journal of Nursing Scholarship, 13,* 71–74.
Hymovich, D. P. (1983). The chronicity impact and coping instrument: Parent ques-
tionnaire. *Nursing Research, 32,* 275–281.
Hymovich, D. P. (1984). Development of the chronicity impact and coping instru-
ment: Parent questionnaire (CICI:PQ) *Nursing Research, 33,* 218–222.
Hymovich, D. P. (1990). Measuring parental coping when a child is chronically ill. In
O. L. Strickland & C. F. Waltz (Eds.), *Measurement of nursing outcomes. Vol.
IV Measuring nursing performance* (pp. 96–117). New York: Springer Publish-
ing Co.
Johnson, D. (1980). Johnson behavioral system model. In J. P. Riehl & C. Roy
(Eds.), *Conceptual models for nursing practice* (pp. 207–290). New York:
Appleton-Century-Crofts.
Khampalikit, S. (1983). The interrelationship between the asthmatic child's de-
pendency behavior, his perception of his illness, and his mother's perception of
his illness. *Maternal Child Nursing Journal, 12,* 221–296.
King, E. H. (1981). Child-rearing practices: Child with chronic illness and well
sibling. *Issues in Comprehensive Pediatric Nursing, 5,* 185–194.
Knafl, K. A., & Deatrick, J. A. (1986). How families manage chronic conditions: An
analysis of the concept of normalization. *Research in Nursing & Health, 9,*
215–222.
Knafl, K. A. & Deatrick, J. A. (1987). Conceptualizing family response to a child's
chronic illness or disability. *Family Relations, 36,* 300–304.

Knafl, K. A., & Deatrick, J. A. (1990). Family management style: Concept analysis and development. *Journal of Pediatric Nursing, 5*, 4–14.

Kruger, S., Shawver, M., & Jones, L. (1980). Reactions of families to the child with cystic fibrosis. *IMAGE: Journal of Nursing Scholarship, 12*, 67–72.

Krulik, T. (1980). Successful 'normalizing' tactics of parents of chronically-ill children. *Journal of Advanced Nursing, 5*, 573–578.

Lazarus, R. S. (1966). *Psychological stress and the coping process*. New York: McGraw-Hill.

Mercer, R. T. (1974). Mothers' responses to their infants with defects. *Nursing Research, 23*, 133–137.

McCubbin, M. A. (1984). Nursing assessment of parental coping with cystic fibrosis. *Western Journal of Nursing Research, 6*, 407–418.

McCubbin, M. A. (1988). Family stress, resources, and family types: Chronic illness in children. *Family Relations, 37*, 203–210.

McCubbin, M. A. (1989). Family stress and family strengths: A comparison of single- and two-parent families with handicapped children. *Research in Nursing & Health, 12*, 101–110.

McCubbin, M. A., & Huang, S. T. T. (1989). Family strengths in the care of handicapped children: Targets for intervention. *Family Relations, 38*, 436–443.

McCubbin, H. I., McCubbin, M. A., Patterson, J., Cauble, A. E., Wilson, L. & Warwick, W. (1983). CHIP-Coping Health Inventory for Parents: An assessment of parental coping patterns in the care of the chronically ill child. *Journal of Marriage & the Family, 45*, 359–370.

McCubbin, H. I., & Patterson, J. M. (1983). The family stress process: The double ABCX model of adjustment and adaptation. *Marriage and Family Review, 6*, 7–37.

McKeever, P. T. (1981). Fathering the chronically ill child. *The American Journal of Maternal Child Nursing (MCN), 6*, 124–128.

Moos, R. H., & Tsu, V. D. (1977). The crisis of physical illness: An overview. In R. H. Moos (Ed.), *Coping with physical illness* (pp. 3–21). New York: Plenum Press.

Moriarty, H. J. (1990). Key issues in the family research process: Strategies for nurse researchers. *Advances in Nursing Science, 12*(3), 1–14.

Murphy, K. M. (1990). Interactional styles of parents following the birth of a high-risk infant. *Journal of Pediatric Nursing, 5*, 33–41.

Murphy, S. (1986). Family study and nursing research. *IMAGE: Journal of Nursing Scholarship, 18*, 170–174.

Orem, D. E. (1971). *Nursing: Concepts of practice* (2nd ed.). New York: McGraw-Hill.

Perrin, J. M. (1985). Introduction. In N. Hobbs & J. M. Perrin (Eds.), *Issues in the care of children with chronic disease* (pp. 1–10). San Francisco: Jossey-Bass.

Pinyerd, B. J. (1983). Siblings of children with myelomeningocele: Examining their perceptions. *Maternal Child Nursing Journal, 12*, 61–70.

Pless, I. B. (1985). Introduction. In N. Hobbs & J. M. Perrin (Eds.), *Issues in the care of children with chronic illness* (pp. 1–10). San Francisco: Jossey-Bass.

Pless, I. B., & Perrin, J. M. (1985). Issues common to a variety of illnesses. In N. Hobbs & J. M. Perrin (Eds.), *Issues in the care of children with chronic illness* (pp. 41–60). San Francisco: Jossey-Bass.

Prescott, P. A. (1987). Multiple regression analysis with small samples: Cautions and suggestions. *Nursing Research, 36*, 130–133.

Rolland, J. S. (1987). Chronic illness and the life cycle: A conceptual framework. *Family Process, 26,* 203–221.

Rolland, J. S. (1988). A conceptual model of chronic and life-threatening illness and its impact on families. In C. S. Chilman, E. W. Nunnally, & F. M. Cox (Eds.), *Chronic illness and disability* (pp. 17–68). Newbury Park, CA: Sage.

Schlomann, P. (1988). Developmental gaps of children with a chronic condition and their impact on the family. *Journal of Pediatric Nursing, 3,* 180–187.

Shapiro, J. (1983). Family reactions and coping strategies in response to the physically ill or handicapped child: A review. *Social Science in Medicine, 17,* 913–931.

Stullenbarger, B., Norris, J., Edgil, A. E., & Prosser, M. J. (1987). Family adaptation to cystic fibrosis. *Pediatric Nursing, 13,* 29–31.

Taylor, S. C. (1980). The effect of chronic childhood illnesses upon well siblings. *Maternal Child Nursing Journal, 9,* 109–116.

Thomas, R. B. (1984). Nursing assessment of childhood chronic conditions. *Issues in Comprehensive Pediatric Nursing, 7,* 165–176.

Thomas, R. B. (1987). Methodological issues and problems in family health care research. *Journal of Marriage and the Family, 49,* 65–70.

Trute, B., & Hauch, C. (1988). Building on family strengths: A study of families with positive adjustment to the birth of a developmentally disabled child. *Journal of Marital and Family Therapy, 14,* 185–193.

Uphold, C. R., & Strickland, O. L. (1989). Issues related to the unit of analysis in family nursing research. *Western Journal of Nursing Research, 11,* 405–417.

Van Cleve, L. (1989). Parental coping in response to their child's spina bifida. *Journal of Pediatric Nursing, 4,* 172–176.

Waechter, E. H. (1977). Bonding problems of infants with congenital anomalies. *Nursing Forum, 16,* 298–318.

PART II

Research on Nursing Care Delivery

Chapter 6

Disaster Nursing

PAULINE KOMNENICH
COLLEGE OF NURSING
ARISONA STATE UNIVERSITY

CAROLYN FELLER
COLLEGE OF NURSING
ARISONA STATE UNIVERSITY

CONTENTS

Historical Perspectives
Definitions and Key Issues
Research Related to Disaster Nursing
Studies in Nursing Education
Personal Accounts of Nurses·
Directions for Future Nursing Research

Although the study of disasters in the social and behavioral sciences is relatively comprehensive and expansive, limited theoretical and research-based information is available in the nursing literature. This review, therefore, represents an effort to examine and summarize the existing literature from the nursing perspective as a way of identifying areas for future nursing research. The approach used to meet that goal was to identify disaster research with a focus on (a) history, (b) definitions and issues, (c) nursing research, and (d) directions for future nursing research.

Much of the literature related to the study of disasters comes from related disciplines with very little research reported by nurses and about nursing. The literature search for this review began with a comprehensive search for data-based articles using key words such as disaster nursing and nursing research of disasters. The initial search brought forth primarily nondata-based articles. Government documents, other pertinent articles, and books also were reviewed and then placed into one of two major categories: (a) education of nurses to prepare them to function effectively during a disaster and (b) personal accounts of nurses' reactions and responses to being involved in a disaster. Categories overlapped at times and articles occasionally fell within both of the categories.

HISTORICAL PERSPECTIVES

Organized efforts to provide disaster relief parallel to some degree the history of medicine dating to the preChristian era. Disaster relief in early societies and under the influence of the Egyptian and Roman Empires is not documented clearly. In the early centuries of the Christian era, there were documented occurrences of large scale disasters but little documentation of responses to these disasters.

One of the most significant large scale and long standing organized disaster relief efforts in contemporary society is that of the Red Cross, which was originally established by Henry Dunant in 1863. Through Clara Barton's efforts, the American Red Cross was established in 1881. A charter from the United States Congress in 1905 required cooperation of the American Red Cross and the government to provide assistance to the sick and wounded in time of war and voluntary relief for victims of disaster (U.S. Congress, 1905). Although the primary emphasis was on assistance to victims, the Red Cross began to recognize the effects of stress on disaster relief workers. Because of the recognition that stress affects workers as well as victims, the American Red Cross instituted training programs for diaster relief workers (Mascelli, 1988).

In addition to the Red Cross, the Department of Defense, and the Federal Emergency Management Agency, church groups and private voluntary organizations such as the National Committee of Voluntary Organizations have organized disaster response activities. With the development of these organized response efforts, documented knowledge about human responses to mass emergencies by victims and caregivers has increased progressively.

According to Drabek (1986), the theoretical foundation of sociological disaster research began in 1920 with a doctoral dissertation by Samuel Prince. Prince (1920) described the organizational responses following a massive chemical explosion in Halifax, Nova Scotia. Prince's case study of this event set the stage for the development of social theory to support future disaster research.

From an historical perspective, the 1950s and 1960s were years in which disaster research moved forward (Drabek, 1986; Kreps, 1984; Lystad, 1988; Quarantelli & Dynes, 1977). Under a contract with the Army Chemical Center, Department of the Army, Fritz and Marks (1954) summarized the disaster studies conducted by the National Opinion Research Center. The Center's studies involved interviews with over 1,000 persons who had experienced one of 70 different major or minor disasters. Key findings of these studies on topics such as panic and convergence behaviors resulted in important policy implications for officials responsible for disaster preparedness (Killien, 1954).

In summarizing the major highlights of disaster studies, Fritz (1961) interpreted disasters, natural or man-made, as a special type of social problem. The growing realization that disasters were a special type of social problem in need of research led to the establishment of the Disaster Research Center at Ohio State University in 1963. This Center served as a major source of contributions to disaster research. The Center, which moved to the University of Delaware in 1985, has continued to focus on a variety of sociological and social science research activities centered around group and organizational preparation for, responses to, and recovery from mass emergencies. The Center also has served as a repository for materials collected by other agencies and researchers, providing materials upon request.

During the 1970s, Mileti, Drabek, and Haas (1975) summarized 627 key disaster study findings into an inventory focusing on the social system being studied. Quarantelli and Dynes (1977) summarized sociological studies completed since World War II. These authors noted the growing interest of researchers from many disciplines in disaster research. However, according to Logue, Melick, and Hansen (1981), there were few university groups in the United States conducting extensive research on disaster. The two groups identified were the Disaster Research Center at Ohio State University, Columbus, and the Natural Hazards Research and Applications Information Center at the University of Colorado, Boulder. Apparently, the only center to conduct epidemiological research of disasters was the Center of Research on the Epidemiology of Disasters at the School of Public Health of Louvain University, Brussels, Belgium. Nationally, the federal agencies that have supported research on the health effects of disaster have been the Center for Environmental Health, Atlanta; the National Institute of Mental Health (Mental Health Disaster Assistance Section); the National Science Foundation and the American Red Cross National Headquarters, Washington, D.C.

Historically, the pattern for research and educational programs related to disasters has been sporadic, tied to some extent to the political milieu within a particular decade. A current extensive inventory of sociological findings regarding human system responses to disaster can be found in Drabek (1986). Drabek capsulizes a growing body of sociological research literature that addresses key issues concerning disasters. The other comprehensive treatise on response to mass emergencies was written by Lystad (1988), who focuses on a wide variety of psychosocial stressors from an interdisciplinary perspective. Both Drabek and Lystad provided in depth reviews of the "state of the art" of disaster research in the social and behavioral science fields. No comparable volumes were found in the nursing literature with the exception of the Laube and Murphy (1985) book.

DEFINITIONS AND KEY ISSUES

Although the intent of the present review was to evaluate nursing research on disasters through a comprehensive search, the literature was limited. One of the problems found in reviewing research conducted in the social sciences as well as in nursing was defining what constitutes a disaster. Definitions ranged from a view of disasters as ". . . extreme situations that result in personal or social readjustment, injury or death" (Wallace, 1956) to definitions focused on disaster as a massive collective stress and disruption of society (Fritz, 1961; Kinston & Rosser, 1974). The Disaster Relief Act of 1974 defined a disaster as any major man-made or natural event of such severity and magnitude to warrant disaster systems (United States Congress, 1974). Logue, Melick, and Hansen (1981) distinguished between man-made and natural disasters in that each type creates a different set of health problems. These authors stressed the need to identify the etiological factors related to increased morbidity and mortality during the various states of a disaster. Since 1981 several authors have discussed public policy issues, issues of definition of disasters, classification, responses, and the value of disaster research (D'Souza, 1984; Kreps, 1984; Pijawka, Cuthbertson, & Olson, 1988; Sims & Baumann, 1985). There is a clear need to develop a workable definition of disasters, to coordinate efforts to maximize the multidisciplinary perspectives, and to address public policy issues.

RESEARCH RELATED TO DISASTER NURSING

One of the earliest attempts at research during a disaster was conducted by Florence Nightingale (1858) during the Crimean War. Nightingale used a set of standards to assess the care provided during the war by comparing the mortality experienced in the British armed forces with that experienced in a civilian population. In doing so, she was able to emphasize to the government the very poor standards of care provided to the public. Although her statistical methods were crude when compared to today's standards, Nightingale was able to bring about substantial reform in the living standards of and health services for the armed forces.

Studies in Nursing Education

The first major attempt to determine whether nurses were prepared to function effectively during a disaster was conducted by Neal (1963) in a National League for Nursing (NLN) pilot project. Under contract to the Federal Civil Defense Agency (which subsequently became the Department of Defense and was later subsumed under several agencies), NLN published the report of this pilot project. Four institutions desirous of developing disaster nursing content for their programs expressed an interest in participating in a series of demonstration projects. The study purpose was to investigate and demonstrate the best preparation for nursing students and hospital nursing staff members in responding to five disaster nursing problems and simulated activities. The purpose was achieved through studies conducted in a hospital nursing service and in educational programs including preparation for practical, diploma, baccalaureate, and graduate nurses.

The four schools of nursing and one hospital nursing service participated in the study from January 27, 1958, to September 6, 1961. Questionnaires were sent to students and faculty in all types of nursing programs throughout the country. These questionnaires were focused on the current status of disaster nursing preparation, the courses offered to prepare nurses for nursing care during disaster, and essential nursing content. A concurrent goal of the project was the development of an achievement test in disaster nursing by the NLN Committee on Nursing Service and Nursing Education in National Defense. Some general conclusions reached in this study were that basic education in nursing included only the fundamental knowledge and skills for effective functioning in disasters. The knowledge and skills identified as essential were considered as part of general nursing and not a clinical specialty. In addition, laboratory experiences were limited, and faculty had only limited preparation in disaster nursing.

Emerging from the conclusions of the Neal (1963) report was a recommendation for interdisciplinary research to determine what functions a nurse must be able to perform in order to provide care in a mass disaster. A second recommendation encouraged definition of the essential body of knowledge necessary to perform the identified functions during a disaster. The remaining recommendations centered around the development of a center for teacher-training for mass disasters with access to military training resources or the Civil Defense Instructor Training Center in existence at that time.

The concerns noted in the Neal (1963) conclusions remain problematic today. First, there are few nursing faculty who have the necessary preparation, experience, or interest in disaster nursing. Second, there is a lack of general agreement as to the essential nursing functions specific to disaster nursing.

Based on the recommendations from the Neal report, common findings by Weaver and Robinson (1967), Ellison (1967), Maule (1967), and Pepper (1967) emphasized the need for nurses to be prepared to function effectively during disasters. Additional research is needed, however, for better definition of the necessary skills specific to disaster nursing. The remaining literature in nursing emphasized personal experiences of nurses involved in disasters, with some effort made to generate knowledge about appropriate nursing actions through these accounts.

Personal Accounts of Nurses

Rayner (1958) was one of the pioneers in studying the responses of health care providers to a disaster. Utilizing a field study approach to investigate nurses' reactions in disasters, she found that nurses generally functioned effectively during disasters due to their task-oriented approach to the situation. They also experienced strong emotional responses. Additionally, she found that the sources of stress for nurses related to the urgency of the situation and the desire to provide excellent care to victims. Problems with organization of care, identification with the victims, and the need to avoid conflicts with other health care workers also were identified as stressors. In this study, the researcher suggested that expectations that health care workers function effec-tively during a disaster cannot be assured due to individual responses to stress. Rayner emphasized that additional research is needed to determine types of responses, factors influencing these responses, and the long-term effects on health care workers.

Patterson (1981) interviewed nurses who were present at the Hyatt Regency Hotel in Kansas City, Missouri, in 1981 just after the second and fourth floor walkways had crashed to the floor killing and maiming about 300 people. The nurses described their immediate and subsequent reactions to the disaster, to the rescue operations, and to the activities during the next few days. They found that the response by the rescue teams and the medical personnel was efficient, but that the staff were emotionally and physically drained.

Demi and Miles (1984) examined nursing leadership following the Hyatt Regency Hotel disaster in 1981. They developed a model of leadership for use as a framework for organizing the data from a case study following the disaster. They obtained data through unstructured interviews of nurses in-volved in the impact and early post impact phases. They found that those nurses who were most effective in leadership roles were those who held formal roles in the disaster response plan and had previous training and experience in disasters. Major concerns identified were the lack of integration of the life flight nurses into the disaster plan and the lack of articulation between the disaster site and the area hospitals. The lack of integration and articulation had a negative impact on the effectiveness of the total plan. Nurses, in general, were excluded from representation on disaster planning and evaluation committees after the disaster.

Miles, Demi, and Mostyn-Aker (1984) expanded the research efforts after the Hyatt Regency disaster and described the physical and emotional reactions as well as the help-seeking behaviors of the rescue workers. The Hopkins Symptom Checklist, the Health Assessment Questionnaire, and the Disaster Personal-Experiential Questionnaire were completed by a convenience sample of 51 rescue workers, nurses, physicians, firemen, emergency medical technicians, and morticians, 2 to 6 months following the disaster. The findings indicated that the distress was serious enough that 60% of the workers sought help from others in order to cope. Although the limitations of a nonrandom selection of subjects, small sample size, and the lack of a comparison group were identified by the researchers, this study provided some interesting and valuable findings that are applicable to future research. Some findings were related to considering the long-term outcomes for rescue workers, the variables that impact on the outcomes, and the use of denial in coping with the distress. The researchers summarized by pointing out that many unmet needs of health care workers related to disasters need to be identified and addressed through research efforts.

The nurses at the Colegio Nacional de Enfermeras, A. C., in Mexico City shared their experiences during the earthquake that occurred on September 19, 1985, in an issue of *The International Nursing Review* ("Mexico Earthquake," 1986). In this same volume two nurses who were part of the health team during the 1985 floods in Puerto Rico related their experiences (Rivera, 1986). Those nurses indicated that the primary problems encountered during the disaster were initial confusion due to a lack of guidelines and a shortage of nurses, doctors, and medications. They recommended that nursing programs include basic guidelines for nurses during disasters and that educational institutions coordinate their efforts with local agencies, such as the American Red Cross and Civil Defense.

Scott (1984), a public health nurse in Invercargill, New Zealand, wrote about Southland's severe flooding. In the United States, Macdonough (1979) shared her two week experiences as an American Red Cross volunteer in Mobile, Alabama, caring for hurricane victims. Ciuca, Downie, and Morris (1977) described the work of the mental health staff after a school bus plunged 50 feet off a bridge to the ground. All of those authors emphasized the need to integrate a mental health team into the hospital disaster plans. Although personal accounts of nurses' experiences during disasters may not be considered scientific research, they offered vivid and rich descriptions that provided direction for future research.

Laube (1973) conducted structured interviews with 27 registered nurses who worked in Corpus Cristi, Texas, during Hurricane Celia in August, 1970. The interview was focused on nine questions concerning personal–social characteristics followed by 19 items related to providing nursing care during a disaster. The interview data indicated that the average nurse had disaster nursing training, held a diploma, and was employed by a hospital. The areas of greatest concern to the nurses were excessive physical demands and concern for their own and their patients' safety. Most of the nurses stated that they coped with their anxiety while on duty and were unaware of any decreased efficiency. When Laube talked with nurses who did not assist with the disaster, most of them indicated their primary responsibility was to be with their families. The major conclusion from Laube's study was that most nurses felt they needed more disaster nursing theory.

Studying post-disaster stress and illness among disaster victims, Murphy (1984; 1989) indicated that many of the past studies reporting both short- and long-term negative health effects as a result of disasters did not use the same measures to assess health outcomes. She also emphasized the need to employ both quantitative and qualitative methods when considering the effects and outcomes of disasters upon victims as well as nurses. Laube and Murphy (1985) have presented a perspective on the present state of the art of research related to disaster recovery. The book was significant because it provides new knowledge and insight into factors that may influence disaster recovery, a framework for nursing interventions, and directions for future research.

Questions remain as to which variables should be studied and for how long after the disaster. Garcia (1985) edited an excellent textbook on disaster nursing. During a graduate research course, she conducted a needs assessment that identified the need and defined the content for the book. Over 250 nurses were asked to identify the types of information they needed to enable them to function more effectively during a disaster. The nurses' concerns focused on 15 topics, and those topics became the chapters for the book. The topics included in the book, which could be used by nurse researchers to guide future studies, were: (a) background and historical perspectives on disasters, (b) skills in rapid field assessment, (c) management and triage at the disaster site, (d) disaster decision-making in the acute care facility, (e) the trauma patient in the disaster setting, (f) the traumatized pregnant patient, (g) management of the irradiated patient, (h) psychological aspects of disaster situations, (i) establishing and managing disaster shelters, (j) functioning in the community health setting, (k) development and design of disaster educational programs, (l) planning mass casualty drills, (m) assessing and using community resources, (n) disaster planning and other administrative aspects of mass casualty situations, and (o) legal implications of nursing practice in a major disaster.

DIRECTIONS FOR FUTURE NURSING RESEARCH

The study of disasters is an important and challenging investigative area for nurse researchers. Scientists in nursing have a responsibility to contribute to basic knowledge of human health responses as well as to develop and test nursing interventions. Research related to nursing roles, responsibilities, and responses of nurses during disasters is sparse and many questions remain unanswered. Do nurses feel prepared to function effectively during a disaster? What are educational institutions including in their curricula to prepare nurses to function effectively during disasters? What variables influence the responses of nurses to disasters?

Because disasters by definition are unexpected and unplanned events, researchers may be unprepared and lack the necessary time to prepare systematic and well-planned studies. Previous research, therefore, becomes important in guiding research efforts in future disaster situations. More rigorous case studies and longitudinal studies of high-risk groups following disasters are needed.

Analytic approaches considering the association between dependent and independent variables could be applied to identify high-risk factors as well as high-risk groups. The majority of researchers have not reflected a conceptual or theoretical basis, with the exception of Demi and Miles (1984) who used a leadership model.

Epidemiological approaches to the study of disasters have been focused primarily on the immediate, postimpact period with the focus on outbreaks of infections and communicable diseases as well as increased mortality that might be directly related to the disaster. Few researchers, however, have considered the long-term effects on mortality and morbidity. Additionally, there may be differences in responses between man-made and natural disasters. Not only may the health problems, both short- and long-term effects, differ, but the variables leading to the health problems may differ. Little comparative research related to nurses' responses to different types of disasters has been carried out, and much of the research lacks precision in identifying etiologic factors and the resulting long-term health effects.

The majority of the research considering the long-term health outcomes indicates that physical and mental health problems should be expected following disasters. However, it is not always clear which variables should be studied, at which time, and for how long. Logue, Melick, and Hansen (1981) point out that it would be helpful for researchers to conceptualize three sets of variables: the dependent variables related to short- and long-term effects, the independent variables related to the experience of being a disaster victim or a health-care worker, and the mediating variables that may modify the effects of the disaster.

Barton (1969) has recommended the use of multivariate analysis to assess the determinants of individual responses that could be helpful in identifying risk factors for various disaster periods. Barton's early recommendation continues to be appropriate today. Research strategies need to include multivariate analysis; more controlled studies with larger, randomly selected samples of target populations and control groups: and long-term follow-up of victims and health care providers.

There is clearly a need for additional research in the area of disaster nursing. The challenge is to define the major variables and determine the indices for measurement. Further research efforts should be focused on identifying the health practices that promote quality of life during and after disasters as well as on developing and testing nursing interventions that promote health.

Collaboration among nurse researchers prepared in the physical, behavioral, and nursing sciences, as well as with researchers in other fields, will be critical to understanding the role of nurses during all phases of a disaster. With their diverse scientific backgrounds, nurse researchers are in key positions to develop integrative research methods. Although a few frameworks were proposed in the literature, very few were tested adequately through research. Nursing interventions during disasters need more extensive investigation. Simulated disaster drills and computer programs could be used to test the responses of nurses as well as their degree of competency. More theoretically oriented research is required to describe further the nursing role during disasters. Future studies of disaster nursing also need to include more manipulated variables and multiple outcome variables measured on more than one occasion. Qualitative research approaches would help capture the disaster response experience as described by nurses and other health care providers.

A number of nursing investigators have made an effort to examine the responses of disaster victims and nurses. Much more research is needed. Hopefully, this review will stimulate nursing investigators to add to the body of knowledge of how best to cope with stressful health care experiences that occur during and following disasters.

REFERENCES

Barton, A. H. (1969). *Communities in disaster: A sociological analysis of collective stress situations*. Garden City, NY: Doubleday.

Ciuca, R., Downie, C. S., & Morris, M. (1977). When a disaster happens. *American Journal of Nursing, 77*, 454–456.

Demi, A. S., & Miles, M. S. (1983). Understanding psychologic reactions to disaster. *Journal of Emergency Nursing, 9*, 11–16.

Demi, A. S., & Miles, M. S. (1984). An examination of nursing leadership following a disaster. *Topics in Clinical Nursing, 6*(1), 63–78.

Drabek, T. E. (1986). *Human systems responses to disaster: An inventory of sociological findings*. New York: Springer-Verlag.

D'Souza, F. (1984). Disaster research—ten years on. *Ekistics, 309,* 496–499.

Ellison, D. (1967). Education for nursing care in disaster. *Nursing Clinics of North America, 2,* 299–307.

Fritz, C. E. (1961). Disasters. In R. K. Merton & R. A. Nisbet (Eds.), *Contemporary social problems* (pp. 651–694). New York: Harcourt.

Fritz, C. E., & Marks, E. S. (1954). The NORC studies of human behavior in disaster. *The Journal of Social Issues, 10,* 26–41.

Garcia, L. M. (Ed.). (1985). *Disaster nursing: Planning, assessment, and intervention*. Rockville, MD: Aspen Systems Corporation.

Killien, L. M. (1954). Some accomplishment and some needs in disaster study. *The Journal of Social Issues, 10,* 66–72.

Kinston, W., & Rosser, R. (1974, December). Disaster: Effects on mental and physical state. *Journal of Psychosomatic Research, 18,* 437–456.

Kreps, G. A. (1984). Sociological inquiry and disaster research. *Annual Review of Sociology, 10,* 309–330.

Laube, J. (1973). Psychological reactions of nurses in disaster. *Nursing Research, 22,* 343–347.

Laube, J., & Murphy, S. A. (Eds.) (1985). *Perspectives on disaster recovery*. Norwalk, CT: Appleton-Century-Crofts.

Logue, J. N., Melick, M. E., & Hansen, H. (1981). Research issues and directions in the epidemiology of health effects of disasters. *Epidemiologic Reviews, 3,* 140–162.

Lystad, M. H. (1988). Perspectives on human response to mass emergencies. In M. H. Lystad (Ed.), *Mental health response to mass emergencies: Theory and practice* (pp. xvii-xxxiv). New York: Brunner/Mazel.

Macdonough, G. P. (1979). Diary of an American Red Cross nurse during a disaster. *Arizona Nurse, 32* (6), 2, 4.

Mascelli, A. T. (1988). American Red Cross disaster services. In M. H. Lystad (Ed.), *Mental health responses to mass emergencies: Theory and practice* (pp. 133–158). New York: Brunner/Mazel.

Maule, H. L. (1967). The nurse in action in disaster. *Nursing Clinics of North America, 2,* 309–324.

Mexico earthquake. (1986). *International Nursing Review, 33,* 125–126.

Miles, M. S., Demi, A. S., & Mostyn-Aker, P. (1984). Rescue workers' reactions following the Hyatt Hotel disaster. *Death Education, 8,* 315–331.

Mileti, D. S., Drabek, T. E., & Haas, E. J. (1975). *Human systems in extreme environments*. Boulder, CO: Boulder Institute of Behavioral Science, University of Colorado.

Murphy, S. A. (1984). Stress levels and health status of victims of a national disaster. *Research in Nursing and Health, 7,* 205–215.

Murphy, S. A. (1989). An exploratory model of recovery from disaster loss. *Research in Nursing and Health, 12,* 67–76.

Neal, M. V. (1963). *Disaster nursing preparation: Report of a pilot project conducted in four schools of nursing and one hospital nursing service*. Washington, DC: National League for Nursing.

Nightingale, F. (1858). *Notes on matters affecting the health, efficiency and hospital administration of the British army*. London: Harrison and Sons.

Patterson, P. (1981). OR staffs respond to the Hyatt casualties. *AORN Journal, 34*, 411–416.

Pepper, E. A. (1967). Disaster: Its meaning for the Canadian nurse. *Nursing Clinics of North America, 2*, 337–348.

Pijawka, D. K., Cuthbertson, B. A., & Olson, R. S. (1988). Coping with extreme hazard events: Emerging themes in natural and technological disaster research. *Omega, 18*, 218–297.

Prince, S. H. (1920). *Catastrophe and social change, based upon a sociological study of the Halifax disaster*. Unpublished doctoral dissertation, Columbia University, New York.

Quarantelli, E. L., & Dynes, R. R. (1977). Response to social crisis and disaster. *Annual Review of Sociology, 3*, 23–49.

Rayner, J. (1958). How do nurses behave in disaster? *Nursing Outlook, 6*, 572–576.

Rivera, A. (1986). Nursing intervention in a disaster. *International Nursing Review, 33*, 140–142.

Scott, K. (1984). Southland's ordeal. *New Zealand Nursing Journal, 77*(4), 8–9.

Sims, G. H., & Baumann, D. D. (1985). Natural hazard research and policy: Time for a gadfly. *The American Statistician, 39*, 358–360.

United States Congress. (1905). *U. S. Congress Act of January 5, 1905, as amended, 36 USC*. Washington, DC: Congress of the United States.

United States Congress. (1974). *Disaster relief act amendments of 1974* (PL. 93-288). Washington, DC: Congress of the United States.

Wallace, A. F. (1956). *Human behavior in extreme situations* (Disaster study number 1, publication 390, p. 1). Washington, DC: National Academy of Sciences, National Research Council.

Weaver, O. J., & Robinson R. C. (1967). Nursing responsibilities in community disaster planning. *Nursing Clinics of North America, 2*, 287–298.

Chapter 7

Nurse Anesthesia Care

MATTILOU CATCHPOLE
SCHOOL OF HEALTH AND HUMAN SERVICES
SANGAMON STATE UNIVERSITY

CONTENTS

Procedures for Review
Postoperative Emetic Symptoms Reduction
Stress in the Perioperative Period
Interactions of Muscle Relaxants and Other Drugs
Postanesthetic Respiratory Tidal Volume
Body Temperature During Surgery
Anesthesia Effects on Physiological Parameters
Physical Characteristics of Equipment and Agents
Future Directions for Research

One of the oldest nursing specialties is that of anesthesiology; nurses have been giving anesthesia for over 100 years. In 1877, Sister Mary Bernard assumed the duties of anesthetist at St. Vincent's Hospital, Erie, Pennsylvania. In 1880, at St. John's Hospital in Springfield, Illinois, the Franciscan Sisters began to give anesthesia and to teach other nurses to give anesthesia. This activity spread over the United States. The result today is a highly skilled nursing specialist (Thatcher, 1984).

The current scope of practice of nurse anesthetists in this country encompasses all the areas and practices that are considered anesthesia-related. This includes pre- and postoperative evaluations and applying, inserting, and interpreting all the monitoring devices used during anesthesia. The choice of anesthetic drugs and how they will be given, as well as the administration of the anesthetic itself, is within the scope of practice of the Certified Registered Nurse Anesthetist (CRNA).

Both physicians and nurses practice anesthesia; many physicians consider anesthesia a practice of medicine. In 1970 the American Medical Association's Committee on Nursing published a statement that "medicine and nursing share many overlapping functions" (Gunn, Nicosia, & Tobin, 1987). Research shows that the quality of patient care is the same whether anesthesia is given by a nurse or a physician (Bechtoldt, 1981; Forrest, 1980).

The present-day nurse anesthetist is a registered nurse (RN) with a baccalaureate degree who has graduated from an accredited nurse anesthesia program of 24 to 36 months, depending on the degree offered. A graduate from an accredited program may take the certifying examination and satisfactory completion allows the nurse to practice as a CRNA. Recertification is required every 2 years.

PROCEDURES FOR REVIEW

Nurse anesthetists have conducted research in two general areas: education and clinical practice. The research reviewed for this chapter was limited to the latter. Other delimitations were: (a) the research was published in the calendar years 1984 to 1987 in refereed journals, and (b) CRNA(s) were sole researcher(s) or their participation was in equal numbers with other researchers. The American Association of Nurse Anesthetists' Education and Research Foundation was contacted for information on CRNA researchers. Three refereed journals, *The AANA Journal, Anesthesiology,* and *Anesthesia, Analgesia* were searched manually.

Using the criteria and selection method described, 26 research articles were found. The general goal(s) of the researchers was one or more of the following: improvement in the quality of patient care, increased patient acceptance of care, and decreased cost of patient care. The studies are reviewed in seven content-focused sections.

POSTOPERATIVE EMETIC SYMPTOMS REDUCTION

Reduction of postoperative nausea and vomiting in patient care would address quality of patient care, increased patient acceptance, and decreased cost of patient care. With the introduction of new procedures such as laparoscopies, the introduction of new anesthetic agents, and an increased concern for cost effectiveness in the patient care areas, more attention has been focused on reduction of emetic symptoms. Many different beliefs concerning the causes and predictors of nausea and vomiting have been expressed over the years. Bellville (1961) postulated that opiates sensitize the vestibular apparatus, causing motion to increase emetic symptoms. Iwamoto and Schwartz (1978) attributed nausea and vomiting to the sense of smell and spatial orientation. Perreault, Normandin, and Plamondon (1982) attributed emetic symptoms to an increase in middle ear pressure. Purkis (1964) found that patients with a history of vomiting prior to admission had a 42.7% incidence of repeat vomiting within the 24-hour post anesthesia period.

McKenzie and Halavan (1987) began a prospective study in 1982 to establish the incidence of postoperative nausea and vomiting in the patient population and to investigate factors that may have caused the nausea and vomiting. The incidence of emetic symptoms was lower than expected. The fentanyl intravenous technique had the lowest incidence rate of 3.02%, followed by isoflurane/nitrous oxide at 3.04%, and halothane/nitrous oxide at 4.35%. The highest incidence rate, 11.6%, occured with enflurane/nitrous oxide. The researchers did not specify the amounts of anesthetic agents or if supplementary drugs were given.

Age and gender were contributing factors of nausea and vomiting. Women had a greater incidence than men, and children had twice the incidence of adults. The best predictor of nausea and vomiting in the recovery room was the presence or absence of emetic symptoms on recovery room arrival. There was minimal increase in nausea and vomiting after medication was given for pain. McKenzie and Halavan concluded that the only information gained that might improve patient care was that pain could be treated with drugs in the recovery room with minimal fear of increasing emetic symptoms. The researchers recognized that the study was limited by a lack of controls on data gathering.

Iwamoto and Schwartz (1978) were among the first to publish on the reduction of nausea and vomiting with the use of droperidol. Iwamoto and Schwartz randomly assigned patients scheduled for eye surgery ($N = 165$) to either a control or a droperidol-treated group. The difference in the incidence of nausea/emesis between the two groups was statistically significant ($p \leq$ .01). Wehner and Gilbert (1985) and Wheaton (1985) compared other drugs to droperidol's ability to act as an antiemetic postoperatively when given in conjunction with anesthetic agents.

Wheaton (1985) compared the effects of droperidol and benzquinamide on two dependent variables, postoperative emetic symptoms and time in the recovery room. The sample consisted of 60 women who were having laparoscopies. Thirty patients received droperidol and 30 received benzquinamide after the induction of anesthesia and intubation. The choice of laparoscopy for the surgical procedure was based on a pilot study of 32 patients who had all types of surgeries. Of the pilot study subjects, only the 18 who had laparoscopies had emetic symptoms. The patients' emetic symptoms were scored according to the Patton Scale of Severity (Patton, Moon, & Dannemiller, 1974). Compared to benzquinamide, droperidol significantly reduced nausea. The time in recovery room was an average of 18 minutes less for the droperidol group, but this difference was not statistically significant.

Wehner and Gilbert (1985) compared preoperative medications given to pediatric patients. Fifty children were randomly selected and then assigned either to a group that received droperidol and glycopyrrolate or to a group that received meperidine and glycopyrrolate. The multiple dependent variables were: (a) time in the recovery room, (b) tranquility, (c) ease of arousal, (d) acceptance of the anesthesia mask, and (e) incidence of nausea and vomiting. The validity and reliability of the tool was not reported. The nurses collecting the data were blind to the group assignments. Group differences were reported as percentages with no statistical tests conducted. The droperidol group showed an improvement in all the dependent variables including emetic symptoms, except for time in the recovery room. The recovery time was increased for the droperidol group. Emetic symptoms were measured only by their presence or absence.

Use of a tested tool to measure nausea and vomiting, and to differentiate between the two, would have improved the study. The results of the study would have been much more persuasive with inferential statistical analysis. Also, their sample included persons with a variety of surgical procedures, introducing more uncontrolled variables. In neither of these two clinical experiments in which other drugs were compared with droperidol, did the investigators control for the type of anesthetic. However, anesthetics were studied in two investigations. Gaskey, Ferriero, Pournaras, and Seecof (1986) studied the postoperative emetic effect of fentanyl, a comparatively new narcotic that has been used both as an adjunct and as the main anesthetic drug. Martin, Williams, and Weis (1987) studied the emetic symptoms of sufentanil, an analogue of fentanyl.

In the Gaskey et al. (1986) research, female patients ($N = 90$) undergoing elective gynecological surgery were divided into three groups. All patients with a history of motion sickness, psychological disorders, or mental handicaps were excluded. All patients received nitrous oxide and oxygen. The comparison groups received fentanyl alone, isoflurane alone, or a combination of both. All patients had either a laparoscopy or laparotomy for tubal ligation. Nausea was recorded only when the patient volunteered the information. The addition of fentanyl significantly increased the incidence of nausea and vomiting. This outcome confirmed the results of other investigators (Hackett, Harris, Plantevin, Pringle, & Avery, 1982; Melnick, Chalasani, & Uy, 1984) but conflicted with findings reported by McKenzie and Halavan (1987) in the first study reviewed. Gaskey et al. (1986) noted that their results would have been improved by checking the patients after they left the recovery room. Rising, Dodgson, and Stein (1985) found that the incidence of vomiting frequently occurred 4 hours after anesthesia.

In the Martin et al. (1987) study, subjects were asked if they thought they would be nauseated after anesthesia. A positive answer did not prevent their inclusion in the group. Subjects were excluded if they said they had a cold, ear infection, or a history of ear infections. All 60 patients were given sufentanil and were divided into 3 supplemental anesthesia groups: nitrous oxide/oxygen; nitrous oxide/oxygen/droperidol; and isoflurane/oxygen. There were 3 types of elective surgical procedures: laparoscopies, arthrotomies, and dental procedures.

In the recovery room, Martin et al. (1987) scored the emetic symptoms according to degree of vomiting severity and vomiting duration, a method similar to that described by Bellville, Bross, and Howland (1959). The patients also were contacted by phone between 24 and 72 hours postoperatively to record their postdischarge emetic symptoms. There were no statistically significant differences in the emetic symptoms between the nitrous oxide/oxygen/droperidol group and the isoflurane/oxygen group. However, emetic symptoms occurred in 6 out of 21 subjects in the former group and in 2 out of 21 subjects in the latter group. Significantly more emetic symptoms occurred when nitrous oxide/oxygen was given without droperidol. Five subjects in the isoflurane/oxygen group who had a previous history of emetic symptoms associated with anesthesia did not have any emetic symptoms.

Statistically signficant differences in awakening and orientation time were found when comparing the nitrous oxide/oxygen/droperidol group and the isoflurane/oxygen group to the nitrous oxide/oxygen group. The group with droperidol took 4 minutes longer to wake than the nitrous oxide/oxygen comparison group. The group receiving isoflurene took 5.5 minutes longer to wake than did the comparison group. However, the researchers questioned the clinical significance of these differences. Because laparoscopy was known to have a high incidence of emetic symptoms at the time the research was done, the type of surgeries should have been controlled or at least reported.

Through the years, nitrous oxide, or laughing gas, the oldest anesthetic agent in use in this country, was considered a benign agent. This assumption has been questioned in a number of studies. Melnick and Johnson (1987) found conflicting reports on the role of nitrous oxide in nausea and vomiting. Alexander, Skupski, and Brown (1984) and Lonie and Harper (1986) found that use of nitrous oxide was associated with an increase in emetic symptoms. Korttila, Hovorka, and Erkola (1987) and Muir, Warner, Buck, Harper, and Kunkel (1986) found that the omission of nitrous oxide did not decrease emetic symptoms.

Melnick and Johnson (1987) studied the effects of nitrous oxide on emetic symptoms and on patient recall during surgery. Sixty female patients having dilatation and curettage, therapeutic abortion, cone biopsy, or laser ablation of vulvar lesions were divided into groups that received nitrous oxide/oxygen and isoflurane and oxygen/isoflurane. Patients with a history of motion sickness or postoperative nausea were eliminated from the study. Patients were evaluated every 15 minutes in the recovery room by a recovery-room nurse who was unaware of the method of anesthesia used. Any patient who complained of pain was given a nonnarcotic oral analgesic. The person who discharged patients from the recovery room was unaware of the anesthetic agents used. Twenty-four hours postoperatively each subject was called and asked about nausea, pain, and recall. There was a statistically significant difference between the groups with the group not receiving nitrous oxide reporting less nausea and vomiting. There were no differences between the two groups in level of consciousness, recall, or pain.

Knowledge about anesthesia-related causes of postoperative emetic symptoms has grown rapidly over the years covered in this review. More research is needed about the relationship between vestibular stimulation and past history of postoperative nausea and vomiting and about the incidence of nausea and vomiting postoperatively in various groups of patients.

STRESS IN THE PERIOPERATIVE PERIOD

Emotional stress causes increased plasma levels of epinephrine and norepinephrine to be secreted by the adrenal gland, with a ratio of four molecules of epinephrine to one molecule of norepinephrine (Dimsdale & Moss, 1980). These catecholamines have a biological half life of 1 to 2 minutes, so measurement of the catecholamine plasma levels is a measurement of acute stress (Guyton, 1981). Because of the risk of increased catecholamine levels to the patient during surgery, efforts have been made to reduce stress with chemicals, knowledge and reassurance, and a change in the patient environment. The sounds of surgery have been pinpointed as a cause of increased patient anxiety and thus are assumed to increase catecholamine levels (Westman & Walters, 1982). Music has been used fairly often and is believed to be successful in reducing anxiety and sedation requirements (Auerbach, 1973).

Bonny and McCarron (1984) reported on the benefits of music as an adjunct to anesthesia. Their sample included 25 patients, 9 of whom had general anesthesia for laparoscopies and 16 of whom received regional anesthesia for a number of different procedures. The study variables included the mean music listening time, the mean surgical time, and anecdotal reports of the patients' acceptance of the music, and reports of reduced anxiety. Inferential statistical analyses as well as the use of psychometrically sound instruments for data collection would have improved this research. With so many uncontrolled variables, a larger sample was needed.

Binnings (1987) studied the effects of auditory distraction on anxiety in ambulatory surgical patients receiving regional anesthesia. This researcher used the State Trait Anxiety Index (STAI) (Spielberger, Gorsuch, & Robertson, 1970) to measure anxiety. The STAI has well-established validity and reliability characteristics. The STAI was given to the patients to measure both trait anxiety and present state of anxiety.

A sample of patients ($N = 40$) was assigned to either the control or experimental group. Patients in the experimental group chose one of four nature tapes to listen to during surgery. The STAI was administered pre-operatively and after one postoperative hour. The effect of auditory distraction was measured by comparing the amount of fentanyl and methohexital (a short-acting barbiturate) requested by patients and patients' anxiety level. Mean anxiety level and the mean amount of methohexital and fentanyl given to the experimental group were significantly less than in the control group. These findings reaffirmed the findings of other investigators.

Gaskey (1987) evaluated the effect of preoperative viewing of a videotape concerning anesthesia on anxiety and knowledge of anesthesia. Forty patients admitted for elective gynecological surgery were assigned to one of two groups. The experimental group was shown the videotape. The STAI and a written anesthesia cognitive test were given to both groups. On admission to the operating room, the patient's level of anxiety was assessed using a synopsis from the Graham and Nemiah (cited in Phippen, 1980) list of physiological signs and symptoms of anxiety. In one to three days after surgery, both groups were interviewed using an investigator-developed, interactive questionnaire based on the Modell-Guerra (1980) model.

There were no differences in STAI scores between the experimental and control groups or in anesthesia cognitive scores. However, Gaskey reported a statistically significant difference in anesthesia knowledge. The investigator also reported more symptoms of anxiety in the patients who did not see the videotape, 47 compared to 23 in the group who did. Thirty-nine patients from both groups stated that the anesthesia care provided was satisfactory enough for them to return to the hospital in the future. The 20 patients who viewed the tape felt it should be shown to other patients.

Gaskey (1987) did not control for potential researcher or sample bias. With both groups having the same cognitive mean, it was difficult to understand how there could be a significant difference in the anesthesia knowledge. A larger sample, data gathered by someone blind to group assignment, and more complete statisitical analyses would have improved this research.

Catchpole (1985) described the effect of preoperative medications on reduction of emotional stress as measured by plasma catecholamine levels. Preoperative medications, usually a narcotic and/or a tranquilizer and a vagal depressant, have had detrimental physiological effects. Many factors in addition to emotional stress can cause changes in catecholamine levels. Catchpole controlled for the effects of position and effects of circadian rhythms, both found to influence cutecholamine levels (Henry, Starman, Johnson, & Williams, 1975).

After a pilot study of 9 patients, Catchpole (1985) chose a sample of 40 patients. Subjects were on no medications known or suspected to have an effect on catecholamine levels and were not expected to go to an intensive care area after leaving the recovery room. Their surgery was scheduled between 7:30 A.M. and 8:30 P.M. Three blood samples were collected under controlled conditions of patient position, venopuncture procedure, and data collection timing and submitted to a comparatively new catecholamine radioenzymatic H^3 assay. The first sample was collected on admission, the second in the preanesthesia room before the preoperative medication was given, and the third 30 minutes after the preoperative medication was given (or not given) in the preanesthesia room. The sample was divided into 5 groups based on the type or presence of preoperative medication. Group 1 ($n = 8$) received narcotics only. Group 2 ($n = 8$) received narcotics and a vagal depressant. Group 3 ($n = 14$) was given narcotics and hydroxyzine. In Group 4 ($n = 6$) various combinations were given: phenothiazine with a narcotic, a vagal depressant and narcotic with phenobarbitol, a vagal depressant and narcotic with hydroxyzine, or diazapam and a vagal depressant. Group 5 ($n = 4$) received no preoperative medication due to human error.

There was no statistically significant difference in epinephrine or norepinephrine levels between the admission blood sample and the sample drawn after arrival in the preanesthesia room. For the third blood sample, there was a statistically significant higher level in the epinephrine levels of the narcotic-only group than in the group that received no premedication. The levels of epinephrine and norepinephrine were lowest in the patients who received no premedication.

It appeared that a narcotic alone was a poor choice if a decrease in emotional stress is the goal. From this research data, the best treatment for emotional stress was a 30-minute stay in a *particular* preanesthesia room. Catchpole's (1985) research would have been greatly strengthened if the investigator had been allowed to select the premedications and plan for a control group who received a placebo.

Topp (1985) described glucose levels in nondiabetic patients in response to the stress of anesthesia and a surgical procedure. Epinephrine has caused an increased amount of glucose to be released in the plasma (Guyton, 1981). Topp studied 11 female patients undergoing various abdominal surgeries. The first blood sample was taken with the first intravenous solution of 5% dextrose in lactated Ringers solution in the operating room or holding area. The subsequent intravenous solutions were lactated Ringers. Blood sugars were tested with a glucometer every 15 minutes after surgery was started. Only two patients maintained a glucose level above normal. The preoperative glucose range fell below the established normal range in 5 patients. The levels of plasma glucose to be expected with the intravenous fluids routinely given to the operative patient have been of concern to anesthesia caregivers. Unfortunately the sample size was very small, as the researcher acknowledged, which detracted from the credibility of the results.

INTERACTIONS OF MUSCLE RELAXANTS AND OTHER DRUGS

Most anesthetics include some sort of muscle relaxant. The shortest acting and most frequently used is succinylcholine. This drug usually causes a series of fleeting muscle contractions of variable duration and severity called fasciculation (Gilman, Goodman, Rall, & Murad, 1985). Some investigators believe that fasciculations cause myalgia postoperatively (Paton, 1959). The most common prevention of succinylcholine-caused fasciculation is a small dose of d-tubocurare approximately 5 minutes before succinylcholine is given (Coppage, Wolfson, & Siker, 1972). Succinylcholine also causes a temporary influx of potassium ion into the plasma in various diseases and injuries (Cooperman, Strobel, & Kennell, 1970; Schaner et al., 1969).

Perry and Wetchler (1984) investigated the effects of diazepam (Valium®) on fasciculation and postoperative myalgia. The sample of 100 outpatients for oral surgery was randomly assigned to four groups. Group 1 received diazepam 5 minutes prior to the induction. Group 2 received d-tubocurare 5 minutes before induction. Group 3 received d-tubocurare with induction taking place as soon as the patient said his eyelids were heavy (an average of 45 seconds). Group 4 received no pretreatment. The severity of fasciculations and recovery time were recorded. The patients were called one day postoperatively and questioned regarding muscular aches and pains.

The severity of fasciculations varied among the groups. Patients who received diazepam and those who received no pretreatment had fasciculations of 60% and 76% respectively. Twelve percent of subjects in Group 2 and 42% in Group 3 fasciculated. Thirty-six percent of the Group 1 patients experienced postoperative myalgia following diazepam pretreatment, but only 16% in Groups 2 and 3 had this complaint following d-tubocurare pretreatment. These findings conflicted with results of other investigators (Eisenberg, Balsley, & Katz, 1977; Fahmy, Malek, & Lappas, 1979; Verma, Chatterji, & Mather, 1978) but were similiar to findings reported by Erkola, Salmenpera, and Tammisto (1980). The researchers stated that there was no statistically significant correlation between the severity of the fasciculations and the severity of postoperative myalgia. Variations in recovery room times were not statistically significant.

Perry and Wetchler (1984) did not report the alpha level chosen as the criterion for statistical significance. Their sample size was adequate, and the possibly confounding variables of different induction techniques and type of surgery were controlled.

Giles (1986) studied the interaction of diazepam and succinylcholine to evaluate its effect on hyperkalemia. He found literature to support that it takes 20 to 30 minutes for diazepam to penetrate the membranes of skeletal muscle cells in vitro (Vyskocil, 1978). Giles (1986) found no studies in which 30 minutes were allowed between the diazepam and the succinylcholine injections.

Giles'sample of 12 rabbits were divided into control and experimental groups that had controlled conditions except that the experimental group received diazepam 30 minutes before the succinylcholine. Serum potassium blood samples were drawn intermittently after the succinylcholine. Both groups showed a statistically significant rise in serum potassium that peaked at 10 minutes. Because the diazepam group had a decrease in potassium during the elapsed 30 minutes, they did not experience hyperkalemia. These results were interesting, but the possibility of a species variation must be kept in mind.

Moore, Ciresi, and Kallar (1986) measured the effects of various drugs on the duration of succinylcholine. They noted controversy in the literature regarding the potentiation of succinylcholine by Innovar®, a fixed-dose combination of droperidol and fentanyl. Collins (1976) denied that potentiation occurred, whereas Lewis (1982) and Wehner (1979) reported that it did. Moore et al. (1986) assigned a sample of 20 patients respectively to one of four groups. One group received no drug, one received droperidol alone, one received fentanyl alone, and one received Innovar. All received the same dose of succinylcholine based on body weight. The muscle was tested for contractibility by tetanic stimulation of the distal ulnar nerve near the wrist every 6 to 10 seconds. No statistically significant difference in the duration of muscle relaxation after succinylcholine was found among the groups. A longer recovery time was seen for all three groups who had received additional drugs: tranquilizer, narcotic, or both than for the groups receiving no additional drugs.

The sample size of 5 in each group was small and the method of assignment was not mentioned. Subjects also received other medications before measurements were made, which could have affected results. The alpha level for statistical significance was not stated.

Sheppard (1986) compared the effects of two long-lasting muscle relaxants, d-tubocurare and pancuronium, on the plasma levels of exogenously given heparin for a sample of 60 gynecologic oncology patients. She monitored the heparin levels as well as the thromboplastin time at 10, 30, and 60-minute intervals after the muscle relaxants were given. There was a significant increase in the heparin levels at 10 and 60 minutes. The thromboplastin time was the same in both groups.

Sheppard's sample was described as 60 patients and then as 56 without any explanation for the loss of subjects. There was no explanation of how the sample was assigned nor mention of the measurements of the dependent variables, heparin and thromboplastin, at 30 minutes. The d-tubocurare dose was based on the patient's body weight. That d-tubocurare causes the release of a greater amount of plasma histamine than other muscle relaxants had been well-established previously. The problem is that histamine release may have caused a wide range of symptoms, from negligible to death-producing (Gilman et al., 1985) and other muscle relaxants were available at the time of this research. Presentation of reassuring information about maintenance of the standard of patient care would have strengthened this research report.

POSTANESTHETIC RESPIRATORY TIDAL VOLUME

Two investigations were done to evaluate methods of increasing postanesthetic respiratory volumes (Drain, 1984; Freeman, 1986). An increase in respiratory volumes can decrease pulmonary complications, including atelectasis. One researcher also noted the decreased cost obtained by earlier removal of the patient from the recovery room.

Freeman (1986) found controversy concerning the effect of doxapram. In several studies researchers showed that doxapram significantly reduced the awakening time by reversing respiratory depression caused by anesthetic agents (Gupta & Dundee, 1973; Riddell & Robertson, 1978; Robertson, MacGregor, & Jones, 1977). In another study, Evers and Dobkin (1967) found that doxapram had no ability to reduce the arousal time from general anesthesia. Freeman (1986) chose a sample of 27 subjects who were undergoing breast biopsy or minor gynecological procedures as outpatients. In this double-blind study, the patients all had identical anesthesia agents, but in varying amounts. Immediately upon extubation, the patients were administered an intravenous bolus of either doxapram (1.5 mg/kg body weight) or normal saline followed by an intravenous infusion of either doxapram or normal saline until full consciousness returned or a time period of 30 minutes elapsed. A coin test of small muscle agility developed by Sikh and Dhulia (1979) was used to assess recovery from anesthesia. There was no significant difference in arousal time between the doxapram group ($n = 12$) and the control group ($n = 14$). Interestingly, there was a significantly higher amount of isoflurane given to patients in the doxapram group.

Freeman (1986) believed that a larger sample might have been helpful in detecting differences. The fact that the 12 patients in the experimental group required an average of 1.11% of isoflurane compared to the control group's 0.78% may have affected the results.

Drain (1984) investigated whether patients who had upper abdominal surgery would increase their functional residual capacity and inspiratory capacity when encouraged to sustain a maximum inspiration or when encouraged to breathe deeply. Fourteen patients were assigned randomly to one of two groups. One group received the deep breathing maneuver, and the other received the maximal inspiration maneuver. Nine of the 14 patients were smokers. No significant difference was found in the percentage prediction of the functional residual capacity between smokers and nonsmokers. Although both groups had a decrease postoperatively from their preoperative functional residual capacity, the decrease was significantly less for the sustained maximal inhalation group. This study would have been improved by a larger sample. Control for the variable of smoking status would have made the results more convincing.

BODY TEMPERATURE DURING SURGERY

A decrease in body core temperature can and usually does occur under both general anesthesia and regional anesthesia, such as a spinal (Morris, 1971; Vaughn & Vaughn, 1981). If the core temperature reaches less than 36°C, there is an increased risk of postoperative complications, including prolonged recovery from anesthesia, increased incidence of venous and pulmonary thrombosis, and increased oxygen consumption caused by shivering (Flacke & Flacke, 1983; Lunn, 1969). The wetness of the surgical area causes a decrease in body temperature resulting from heat lost through vaporization (Gravenstein & Paulus, 1982).

Radel, Fallacaro, & Sievenpiper (1986) described the effects of a warming vest and cap during lower-extremity orthopedic surgical procedures under general anesthesia. Thirty patients were randomly assigned to one of three groups. Group 1 (the control group) was covered with a patient gown and two cotton blankets. Patients in Group 2 (passive heat loss protection) were covered with two cotton shirts, a cotton skull cap, and two cotton blankets. Patients in Group 3 (active heat loss protection) had the same items as in Group 2 plus a circulating fluid warming vest and cap made of material used to construct warming blankets. The vest fluid was kept at 38°C, and intravenous fluid was heated to 37°C. No significant differences were found among the three groups for the first 60 minutes of anesthesia. A significant difference was found between the mean temperatures in the control group and the active (vest and cap) group after 120 minutes, at which time only 4 subjects remained in each of these groups.

It is unfortunate that Radel et al.'s sample size was not large enough to assure sufficient numbers in each group to continue to gather data as the length of surgery increased. Heating the intravenous fluids is not a routine practice to counteract body temperature reduction, and perhaps the differences between the groups would have been greater if the fluid had not been heated.

Lombardi-Garner (1985) studied the effect of heating and humidifying anesthetic gases on body temperature. Thirty female patients were assigned to either the experimental group in which the anesthetic gases were heated and humidified or to a comparison group in which they were not. Ventilation volume and room temperature were controlled. Although the group with the heated and humidified gases had a slightly higher temperature, the difference was not significant statistically. She did not state an alpha level for statistical significance. The researcher's conclusions that warming and humidifying the anesthetic gases were important in maintaining body temperature may be true but were not supported by the results of this study.

ANESTHESIA EFFECTS ON PHYSIOLOGICAL PARAMETERS

Kochansky (1986) investigated cardiological responses to diazepam/nitrous oxide anesthesia and surgical stress when intravenous lidocaine was used in a sample of patients with known arteriosclerotic cardiovascular disease. Sample size was not mentioned. All patients, if their condition permitted, received diazepam orally and glycopyrrolate intramuscularly one hour before arrival in the operating room. Each patient was given diazepam and lidocaine intravenously on a body weight dosage prior to the sodium pentothal induction. Cardiovascular parameters were measured during intubation. The investigator found a decreased heart rate during the lidocaine injection. The mean arterial pressure decreased. The decrease in the cardiac index was statistically significant, and the pulmonary capillary wedge pressure increased clinically but not at a statistically significant level. A statistically significant decrease was noted in the left ventricular stroke work index.

Kochansky (1986) concluded that lidocaine could attenuate stress responses to anesthesia induction and intubation, an unwarranted conclusion because of the lack of a control group. All of the responses cited were clinically undesirable. The sample size was unknown, and a control or comparison group was not used. Another weakness in this research was variation in pretreatment of the patients for unstated reasons.

Moyer (1987) assessed the reliability of the pulmonary wedge pressure in measuring left atrial pressure. The sample of 24 patients with myocardial vascularization was divided into two groups: those having good left ventricular function and those with poor function, according to criteria listed in the article. In the patients with good function, the correlation coefficients between pulmonary wedge and left atrial pressures ranged from 0.61 to 0.89. However, in the group with poor left ventricular function, the correlation coefficients ranged from -0.34 to 0.59. In the patients with cardiac failure, pulmonary wedge pressure was an unreliable estimate of left atrial pressure. This replication study was of value given that differences of opinion have been reported concerning the reliability of pulmonary wedge pressure as an indicator of left atrial pressure (Falicov & Resnekov, 1970; Lappas, Lell, Gabel, Civetta, & Lowenstein, 1973; Murphy, 1958; Walston & Kendall, 1973).

Another physiological parameter affected by anesthesia is the intraocular pressure. A problem with open globe ocular surgery has been the need to keep the intraocular pressure at or below normal to prevent the expulsion of vitreous and resultant loss of vision (Duncalf, 1975). Olinder, Smith, Weaver, and Orr (1984) selected 30 patients scheduled for surgery who met the study criteria and assigned them to receive isoflurane, enflurane, or halothane. Intraocular pressure was measured preoperatively and after induction with sodium pentothal. After the postinduction measurement, patients received the inhalant; intraocular pressure was measured at 10, 20, and 30-minute intervals. There were no significant differences among the three groups. The value of this research was the comparison of isoflurane, a newer anesthetic, with well-researched inhalants that have been in use a longer period of time.

Breckenridge (1985) used 24 rabbits to evaluate the effects of clonidine on tachyphylaxis when given in conjunction with sodium nitroprusside, a peripheral vasodilator used to induce hypotension. It has been desirable to reduce the amount of sodium nitroprusside given to gain the needed effect because of the cyanide metabolite of the drug (Gilman et al., 1985). Three groups of eight rabbits each received sodium nitroprusside, two of which also received clonidine at two different doses. Halothane was the anesthetic for the three groups. The author concluded that pretreatment with clonidine reduced the amount of sodium nitroprusside needed. The data were submitted to inferential statistical analysis, but the alpha level chosen for significance was not stated. The groups did not have similar base/mean arterial pressures, and approximately half of the rabbits became acidotic and were given sodium bicarbonate. Unfortunately, how this half of the sample was distributed between groups was not identified. A larger sample or perhaps only two groups, likely would have made less pretest variance between groups.

Rector, DeNuccio, and Alden (1987) compared cocaine, oxymetazoline, and saline for nasotracheal intubation. Epistaxis reduction during nasal intubation was the researchers' goal. Similar research was done with cocaine and other vasoconstrictor/local anesthetic combinations (Gross, Hartigan, & Schaffer, 1984; Mitchell, Lecky, & Levy, 1984). Cocaine has remained unique among local anesthetics in causing vasoconstriction. Vasoconstriction of nasal mucous membranes just before the nasoendotracheal tube is inserted is considered desirable, even when the patient is already anesthetized. The resulting increased diameter of the nares has been assumed to decrease the amount of bleeding; bleeding that could result in increased blood in the respiratory passages and/or lungs. Alternatives to cocaine, a regulated narcotic, would be desirable because cocaine may cause significant arrhythmias (Orr & Jones, 1968) and may increase anesthetic requirements during general anesthesia (Stoelting, Creasser, & Martz, 1975).

The double-blind study was designed by Rector et al. (1987) using cocaine 10%, oxymetazoline 0.5%, and normal saline in numbered vials with the same volume of solution. The sample was composed of 36 patients having impacted molars extracted under general anesthesia. Any patient presumed to have predisposing factors to epistaxis was excluded from the sample. The randomly designated medication was sprayed by someone other than the intubator, who was out of the room. Induction of anesthesia was standardized, and epistaxis was measured prior to surgery and after intubation. No statistically significant differences were found among the three groups. This result was not expected by the researchers, who concluded that the alternative to cocaine either could be nothing or the relatively benign oxymetazoline. Rector et al. recommended further research before cocaine be abandoned. Replication of those findings will be necessary before clinicians give up this deeply ingrained practice (Gross et al., 1984; Mitchell et al., 1984; Verlander & Johns, 1981). Finding similiar results should lead to safer clinical practice without cocaine spray.

PHYSICAL CHARACTERISTICS OF EQUIPMENT AND AGENTS

Kelly and Biddle (1987) investigated anesthesia circuit filters employed universally to prevent pathogens or particulates from contaminating the patient and the apparatus. Five from each of 6 brands of filters available were tested. The authors tested the efficacy of the filters using flow rates from 5 liters per minute to 117 liters per minute. They also measured the amount of resistance the filters added to the patients' respiratory circuit. There was no variation of performance at the same liter flow rate among the 5 filters for any of the six brands. There were differences in the filtering capability at different flow rates and differences between different types of filters. The authors suggested that their results be added to the package insert accompanying the filters.

Kelly and Biddle's analysis included no use of inferential statistics. Valuable new information was gained, but more research is needed using lower flow rates because results did vary with different flow rates. Anesthesia is given at lower flow rates, as low as 0.5 liters per minute in closed-circuit anesthesia.

Biddle and Landess (1986) have been concerned with patient acceptance of an inhalational agent when not preceded by an intravenous drug. The patient must accept the agent enough to breathe it, preferably without force being used. Children are more likely than adults to receive an inhalant without an intravenous drug first. Anesthesia caregivers generally have believed that halothane should be employed preferentially over enflurane or isoflurane because it is the least irritating and least likely to cause reflex activity of the patient's respiratory tract such as coughing, breath-holding, and laryngo-spasms (Stoelting & Miller, 1989).

In their clinical practice these investigators had not found a difference in patient acceptance of these inhalational agents if preceded by 70% nitrous oxide and 30% oxygen for a period of 30 to 60 seconds. Controlled studies were not found, but there were many articles in which great differences in the patient acceptance of these three inhalants were described (Eger, 1984; Stoelting & Miller, 1989). These researchers hoped to validate that patient acceptance need not affect choice of agents.

The Biddle and Landess sample consisted of 300 nonmedical adult individuals, 178 men and 122 women between the ages of 17 and 41 who were in excellent health and free from olfatory deficits. A double-blind study was done. Each subject was asked to sniff briefly the three randomly ordered flasks with a 60-second rest period between presentation of each flask. They first were asked to evaluate the smell, and then were asked which smell they would prefer while being anesthetized. There were no statistically significant differences in the responses of the subjects. The smells of the anesthetics were disliked equally. Biddle and Landess (1986) call to attention the fact that extrapolation to a sick adult population or to a pediatric population may be inappropriate. The sample size was appropriate. This research should be continued in the clinical area with pediatric and adult patients.

FUTURE DIRECTIONS FOR RESEARCH

The majority of the research reports reviewed reflected the investigators' concern for quality of patient care, acceptance of care by the patient, or reduction of patient care cost in terms of length and type of care required. There should be improvement in the quality of the investigators. Research methods and reports of the results of research done by nurse anesthetists should improve as more of the Nurse Anesthesia Programs move to the Master's level. All programs are to be at this level, or greater, by 1998.

ACKNOWLEDGMENTS

My thanks to Jack Kless, CRNA for helping in the search for research in which CRNAs participated. My thanks also to June Hamilton and Joseph Gudgel in the preparation of this manuscript and Carrie O'Rourke for editing the final draft.

REFERENCES

Alexander, G. D., Skupski, J. N., & Borwn, E. M. (1984). The role of nitrous oxide in postoperative nausea and vomiting. *Anesthesia and Analgesia, 63,* 175.
Auerbach, S. (1973). Trait-State Anxiety and adjustment to surgery. *Journal Consultant and Clinical Psychology, 40,* 264–271.
Bechtoldt, A. (1981). Committee on anesthesia study anesthesia-related deaths: 1969–1976. *North Carolina Medical Journal, 42,* 253–259.
Bellville, J. W. (1961). Postanesthestic nausea and vomiting. *Anesthesiology, 22,* 773–780.
Bellville, J. W., Bross, I. D. J., & Howland, W. S. (1959). A method for clinical evaluation of antiemetic agents. *Anesthesiology, 20,* 753–760.
Biddle, C., & Landess, B. (1986). An analysis of the subjective pungencies of inhalational anesthetics. *AANA Journal, 54,* 433–435.
Binnings, E. B. (1987). The effect of an auditory distraction on anxiety in ambulatory surgical patients experiencing regional anesthesia. *AANA Journal, 55,* 333–335.
Bonny, H., & McCarron, N. (1984). Music as an adjunct to anesthesia in operative procedures. *AANA Journal, 52,* 55–57.
Breckenridge, H. K. (1985). The effect of clonidine on the reduction of tachyphylaxis. *AANA Journal, 53,* 476–479.
Catchpole, M. (1985). Do preoperative medications reduce emotional stress as measured by plasma catecholamine levels? *AANA Journal, 53,* 327–331.
Collins, V. J. (1976). *Principles of anesthesiology,* (2nd ed.). Philadelphia: Lea and Febiger.

Cooperman, L. H., Strobel, G. E., & Kennell, E. M. (1970). Massive hyperkalemia after administration of succinylcholine. *Anesthesiology, 32,* 161–164.

Coppage, W. M., Wolfson, B., & Siker, E. S. (1972). Precurarization and dose of succinylcholine. *Anesthesiology, 37,* 664–665.

Dimsdale, J. E., & Moss, J. R. (1980). Plasma catecholamine in stress and exercise. *Journal of the American Medical Association, 243,* 340–342.

Drain, C. B. (1984). Comparison of two inspiratory maneuvers on increasing lung volumes in postoperative upper abdominal surgical patients. *AANA Journal, 52,* 379–388.

Duncalf, D. (1975). Anesthesia and intraocular pressure. *Bulletin of the New York Academy of Medicine, 51,* 374–381.

Eger, E. I. (1984). Current controversies concerning enflurane and isoflurane. In P. G. Barash (Ed.) *ASA refresher courses in anesthesiology* (pp. 1–6). Philadelphia: J. B. Lippincott.

Eisenberg, M., Balsley, S., & Katz, R. L. (1977). Effects of diazepam on succinylcholine induced myalgia, potassium increase, creatinine phosphokinase elevation, and relaxation. *Anesthesia and Analgesia, 58,* 314–317.

Erkola, O., Salmenpera, M., & Tammisto, T. (1980). Does diazepam pretreatment prevent succinylcholine induced fasciculations? A double blind comparison of diazepam and tubocurarine pretreatments. *Anesthesia and Analgesia, 59,* 932–934.

Evers, W., & Dobkin, A. B. (1967). Influence of doxapram hydrochloride on recovery from thiopental anesthesia. *New York Medical Journal, 67,* 3236–3241.

Fahmy, M. R., Malek, N. S., & Lappas, D. G. (1979). Diazepam prevents some adverse effects of succinylcholine. *Clinical Pharmacology and Therapeutics, 26,* 395–398.

Falicov, R. E., & Resnekov, L. (1970). Relationships of the pulmonary artery end-diastolic pressure to the left ventricular end diastolic and mean filling pressures in patients with and without left ventricular dysfunction. *Circulation, 42,* 65–73.

Flacke, J. W., & Flacke, W. E. (1983). Inadvertent hypothermia: Frequent, insidious, and often serious. *Seminars in Anesthesia, 2,* 183–196.

Forrest, W. H. (1980). Outcome—The effect of the provider. In R. Hirsch (Ed.), *Health care delivery in anesthesia,* (pp. 137–140). Philadelphia: George F. Stickley Co.

Freeman, D. J. (1986). The effectiveness of doxapram administration in hastening arousal following general anesthesia in outpatients. *AANA Journal, 54,* 16–20.

Gaskey, N. J. (1987). Evaluation of the effect of a pre-operative anesthesia videotape. *AANA Journal, 55,* 341–345.

Gaskey, N. J., Ferriero, L., Pournaras, L., & Seecof, J. (1986). Use of fentanyl markedly increases nausea and vomiting in gynecological short stay patients. *AANA Journal, 54,* 309–311.

Giles, H. W. (1986). The effect of diazepam in the prevention of succinylcholine-induced hyperkalemia. *AANA Journal, 54,* 21–22.

Gilman, A. G., Goodman, L. S., Rall, T. W., & Murad, F. (1985). *The pharmacological basis of therapeutics* (7th ed.). New York: MacMillan.

Gravenstein, J. S., & Paulus, D. A. (1982). *Monitoring practice in clinical anesthesia.* Philadelphia: J. B. Lippincott.

Gross, J. B., Hartigan, M. L., & Schaffer, D. W. (1984). A suitable substitute for 4% cocaine before blind nasotracheal intubation: 3% lidocaine—0.25% phenylephrine nasal spray. *Anesthesia and Analgesia, 63,* 915–918.

Gunn, I. P., Nicosia, J., Tobin, M. (1987). Anesthesia: A practice of nursing. *AANA Journal, 55,* 98–100.

Gupta, P. K., & Dundee, J. W. (1973). Hastening of arousal after general anaesthesia with doxapram hydrocholide. *British Journal of Anaesthesia, 45,* 493–496.

Guyton, A. C. (1981). *Textbook of Medical Physiology* (7th ed.). Philadelphia: Saunders.

Hackett, G. H., Harris, M. N. E., Plantevin, H. M., Pringle, D. B., & Avery, A. J. (1982). Anaesthesia for outpatient termination of pregnancy. *British Journal of Anaesthesia, 54,* 865–870.

Henry, D. P., Starman, B. J., Johnson, D. G., & Williams R. H. (1975). A sensitive radioenzymatic assay for norepinephrine in tissue and plasma. *Life Sciences, 16,* 375–378.

Iwamoto, K., & Schwartz, H. (1978). Antiemetic effect of droperidol after ophthalmic surgery. *Archives of Opthamology, 96,* 1378–1379.

Kelly, M. E., & Biddle, C. (1987). A qualitative analysis of anesthesia circuit filters: Resistance and penetrance characteristics. *AANA Journal, 55,* 233–236.

Kochansky, S. W. (1986). Cardiovascular responses to anesthesia and surgical stress when intravenous lidocaine is used as an adjunct to diazepam-nitrous oxide anesthesia for vascular surgery. *AANA Journal, 54,* 199–200.

Kortila, K., Hovorka, J., & Erkola, O. (1987). Omission of nitrous oxide does not decrease the incidence or severity of emetic symptoms after isoflurane anesthesia. *Anesthesia and Analgesia, 66,* S98.

Lappas, D., Lell, W. A., Gabel, J. C., Civetta, J. M., & Lowenstein, E. (1975). Indirect measurement of left atrial pressure in surgical patients' pulmonary capillary wedge and pulmonary artery diastolic pressures compared with left atrial pressure. *Anesthesiology, 38,* 394–398.

Lewis, R. A. (1982). A consideration of prolonged succinylcholine paralysis with Innovar. Is the cause droperidol or fentanyl? *AANA Journal, 50,* 55–59.

Lombardi-Garner, G. (1985). The effects of the heating and humidifying of anesthetic gases on the maintenance of body temperature. *AANA Journal, 53,* 473–476.

Lonie, D. S., & Harper, N. J. N. (1986). Nitrous oxide anaesthesia and vomiting. *Anaesthesia, 41,* 703–707.

Lunn, H. F. (1969). Observations on heat gain and loss in surgery. *Guy Hospital Reports, 118,* 117–127.

Martin, J., Williams, D., & Weis, F. R. (1987). Comparison of three anesthetic techniques on emetic symptoms using sufentanil for outpatient surgery. *AANA Journal, 55,* 245–249.

McKenzie, S. A., & Halavan, J. (1987). An investigation into post-anesthesia nausea and vomiting in a community hospital-based anesthesiology practice. *AANA Journal, 55,* 427–433.

Melnick, B. M., Chalasani, J., & Uy, N. T. L. (1984). Comparison of enflurane, isoflurane, and continuous fentanyl infusion for outpatient anesthesia. *Anesthesiology Review, 11*(7), 36–39.

Melnick, B. M., & Johnson, L. S. (1987). Effects of eliminating nitrous oxide in outpatient anesthesia. *Anesthesiology, 67,* 982–984.

Mitchell, R. L., Lecky, J. H., & Levy, W. J. (1984). A comparison of nasal spray with lidocaine/phenylephrine, and saline for nasal intubation. *Anesthesiology, 61,* A217.

Modell, J. G., & Guerra, F. (1980). *Emotional and psychological responses to anesthesia and surgery* (1st ed.). New York: Grune & Stratton.

Moore, G. B., Ciresi, S., & Kallar, S. (1986). The effect of innovar versus droperidol or fentanyl on the duration of action of succinylcholine. *AANA Journal, 54,* 130–136.

Morris, R. H. (1971). Operating room temperature and the anesthetized, paralyzed patient. *Archives of Surgery, 102,* 95–97.

Moyer, M. K. (1987). Pulmonary wedge pressure does not accurately reflect left atrial pressure in patients with severe left ventricular dysfunction. *AANA Journal, 55,* 336–340.

Muir, J. J., Warner, M. A., Buck, C. F., Harper, J. V., & Kunkel, S. E. (1986). The role of nitrous oxide in producing postoperative nausea and vomiting. *Anesthesiology, 65,* A461.

Murphy, J. P. (1958). Inaccuracy of wedge pressure in animals estimated by venous and arterial catheterization. *Circulation, 17,* 199–202.

Olinder, P. J., Smith, R. B., Weaver, J., & Orr, M. D. (1984). Intraocular pressure following inhalation anesthesia and sodium thiopental. *AANA Journal, 52,* 373–377.

Orr, D., & Jones, I. (1968). Anaesthesia for laryngoscopy—A comparison of the cardiovascular effects of cocaine and lidocaine. *Anaesthesia, 23,* 194–202.

Paton, W. D. M. (1959). The effects of muscle relaxants other than muscular relaxation. *Anesthesiology, 20,* 453–463.

Patton, C. M., Moon, M. R., & Dannemiller, F. J. (1974). The prophylactic antiemetic effect of droperidol. *Anesthesia and Analgesia, 53,* 361–364.

Perreault, L., Normandin, N., & Plamondon, L., Blain, R., Rouseau, P., Girard, M., & Forget, G. (1982). Middle ear pressure variations during nitrous oxide and oxygen anaesthesia. *Canadian Anaesthetist's Society Journal, 29,* 428–434.

Perry, J., & Wetchler, B. V. (1984). Effects of diazepam pretreatment of succinylcholine on fasciculation or postoperative myalgia in outpatient surgery. *AANA Journal, 52,* 48–50.

Phippen, M. L. (1980). Nursing assessment of preoperative anxiety. *Association of Operating Room Nurses Journal, 31,* 1019–1026.

Purkis, I. E. (1964). Factors that influence postoperative vomiting. *Canadian Anaesthetist's Society Journal, 11,* 335–353.

Radel, T. J., Fallacaro, M. D., & Sievenpiper, T. (1986). The effects of a warming vest and cap during lower extremity orthopedic surgical procedures under general anesthesia. *AANA Journal, 54,* 486–489.

Rector, F. T. R., DeNuccio, D. J., & Alden, M. A. (1987). A comparison of cocaine, oxymetazoline, and saline for nasotracheal intubation. *AANA Journal, 55,* 49–54.

Riddell, P. L., & Robertson, G. S. (1978). Use of doxapram as an arousal agent in outpatient general anaesthesia. *British Journal Anaesthesia, 50,* 921–924.

Rising, S., Dodgson, M. S., & Steen, P. A. (1985). Isoflurane v. tentanyl for outpatient laparoscopy. *ACTA Anaethesiology Scandinavia, 29,* 251–255.

Robertson, G. S., MacGregor, D. M., & Jones, C. J. (1977). Evaluation of doxapram for arousal from general anaesthesia in outpatients. *British Journal Anaesthesia, 49,* 133–140.

Schaner, P. J., Brown, R. L., Kirksey, T. D., Gunther, R. C., Ritchey, C. R., & Gronert, G. A. (1969). Succinylcholine induced hyperkalemia in burned patients. *Anesthesia and Analgesia, 48,* 764–770.

Sheppard, M. L. (1986). Does the use of d-tubocurarine decrease coagulability in patients given low dose preoperative heparin prophylaxis? *AANA Journal, 54,* 152, 169.

Sikh, S. S., & Dhulia, P. N. (1979). Recovery from general anesthesia—simple and comprehensive test for assessment. *Anesthesia and Analgesia, 58,* 324–326.

Spielberger, C. D., Gorsuch, R. I., & Robertson, D. (1970). *Manual for the State Trait Anxiety Inventory*. Palo Alto: Palo Alto Publishing.

Stoelting, R. K., Creasser, C. W., & Martz, R. C. (1975). Effect of cocaine administration on halothane MAC in dogs. *Anesthesia and Analgesia, 54,* 422–424.

Stoelting, R. K., & Miller, R. D. (1989). *Basics of anesthesia* (2nd ed.). New York: Churchill Livingstone.

Thatcher, V. S. (1984). *History of anesthesia with the emphasis on the nurse specialist*. New York: Garland.

Topp, D. (1985). The nondiabetic's blood glucose tolerance to the stress of surgery. *AANA Journal, 53,* 338–341.

Vaughn, M. S., & Vaughn, R. W. (1981). Postoperative hypothermia. *Surgical Rounds, 4,* 34–38.

Verlander, J. M., & Johns, M. E. (1981). The clinical use of cocaine. *Otolaryngologic Clinic of North America, 14,* 521–531.

Verma, R. S., Chatterji, S., & Mather, N. (1978). Diazepam and succinylcholine induced muscle pains. *Anesthesia and Analgesia, 57,* 295–297.

Vyskocil, F. (1978). Effects of diazepam on the frog neuromuscular junction. *European Journal of Pharmacology, 48,* 117–124.

Walston, A., & Kendall, M. E. (1973). Comparison of pulmonary wedge and left atrial pressure in man. *American Heart Journal, 86,* 159–164.

Wehner, R. J. (1979). A case study: The prolongation of Anectine® effect by Innovar. *AANA Journal, 47,* 576–599.

Wehner, R. J., & Gilbert, D. H. (1985). Premedication of children with droperidol–glycopyrrolate versus meperidine–glycopyrrolate: Results of a blind study. *AANA Journal, 53,* 504–507.

Westman, J. C., & Walters, J. R. (1982). Noise and stress: A comprehensive approach. *Environmental Health Perspectives, 41,* 291–309.

Wheaton, N. E. (1985). Comparison of benzquinamide hydrochloride and droperidol in preventing postoperative nausea and vomiting following general outpatient anesthesia. *AANA Journal, 53,* 322–326.

PART III
Research on Nursing Education

Chapter 8

Occupational Health Nursing Education

BONNIE ROGERS

SCHOOL OF PUBLIC HEALTH

UNIVERSITY OF NORTH CAROLINA—CHAPEL HILL

CONTENTS

This review includes research on occupational health nursing education. Procedures and methodological issues related to the review, research on undergraduate and graduate education, trends in occupational health nursing education, and future research regarding conceptual development of the field are addressed.

Occupational health nursing includes the application of nursing principles in promoting the health of workers and maintaining a safe and healthful workplace (AAOHN, 1988). It requires a synthesis of knowledge in related fields of study such as toxicology, industrial hygiene, safety, public health sciences, and human behavior. Increasingly, more emphasis has been placed on health promotion, health protection, and disease prevention aspects of practice. Formerly called industrial nursing, the term occupational health nursing is now used to reflect the broader scope of practice in the field. The term industrial nursing will be used during the historically relevant segment of this chapter.

In conducting this review, several approaches were utilized for the retrieval of relevant information and research literature. Computerized searches were conducted to retrieve information from 1970 to 1989. Data bases searched included: MEDLINE, CINAHL, ERIC, Excerpta Medica, Dissertation Abstracts, Federal Research in Progress, and NIOSHTIC. The following key words were used: occupational health nursing, industrial health nursing, public health nursing, community health nursing, undergraduate nursing education, graduate nursing education, curriculum, and research. All terms that did not include "occupational health or industrial health" were cross-referenced to these terms (e.g., public health nursing in industry and occupational health settings) in order to exclude irrelevant documents.

A manual search was conducted in the Cumulative Index to Nursing and Allied Health (1970–1989), and in specific journals relevant to the topic including the *Occupational Health Nursing Journal* (1975–1985), *AAOHN Journal* (1986–1990), and *Public Health Nursing* (1985–1990). In addition, the Public Health Nursing Library at the University of North Carolina at Chapel Hill has several documents from the National League for Nursing (NLN) and American Nurses' Association (ANA) that provided historical information related to educational development and trends in occupational health nursing. Relevant historical documents from the American Association of Occupational Health Nurses (AAOHN) Library related to occupational health nursing education also were reviewed.

Criteria for inclusion were that studies be reported in English and be data-based; literature with relevant historical underpinnings also was reviewed. A total of 17 research reports and 9 related historical documents were reviewed. There are several reasons for the paucity of research in this area: (a) lack of understanding of the practice of occupational health nursing within the mainstream of nursing; (b) relatively little occupational health nursing content in nursing curricula; (c) few nursing faculty interested in the field of occupational health nursing; and (d) insufficient numbers of occupational health nurse educators and researchers.

METHODOLOGICAL ISSUES

Limitations of the studies reviewed require that caution be used in the application of the findings to educational programs. As indicated above, occupational health nursing practice involves the synthesis of principles from nursing, public health, and other disciplines. However, several researchers used a task-oriented approach to identify practice elements rather than a clearly identified conceptual approach to curriculum derivation. This is not surprising given the relative newness of research in occupational health nursing.

All studies reviewed involved some form of descriptive research, with survey designs employed most frequently. One study was national in scope, one regional, two statewide, and all others local. Excepting where total populations were used, sample selection was mostly purposive or by convenience, and sample sizes often were small.

In all but one study, instruments were developed by the authors. Content validity either was reported explicitly or implied; however, no other types of validity or reliability were reported. Lack of instrument testing may have been due to the general lack of research conducted in occupational health nursing prior to the 1980s. Data were analyzed mostly using descriptive and nonparametric statistical techniques, which is consistent with the type and state of the research.

UNDERGRADUATE EDUCATION

Education for industrial nursing in the early 1900s was influenced by the development of worker's compensation laws in 1911 and World War I. As industrial nursing began to proliferate, coursework specific to nursing in industrial settings was needed. In 1917 Boston College provided the first course "Industrial Services for Nurses," which was offered as 2-hour lectures twice weekly for 16 weeks (McGrath, 1946). The course was offered annually for 5 years and included content related to injuries and illness care, labor laws, economics, and communicable disease treatment and prevention.

In the 1930s the impetus for improvement in industrial nursing education was strong. The American Public Health Association (APHA) and the National Organization of Public Health Nursing (NOPHN) conducted a study of the duties and functions of 85 nurses working in 42 companies in the late 1930s. The results indicated a lack of uniform nursing practices and standards, lack of awareness and underutilization of community resources by industrial nurses, and inadequate courses to prepare nurses to practice in industrial settings (NOPHN, 1941). These findings were supported by a similar study conducted by the Division of Industrial Hygiene, United States Public Health Service and the APHA in 1944 (Whitlock, Tasko, & Kohl, 1944), which prompted the American Association of Industrial Nurses (AAIN) (now the American Association of Occupational Health Nurses) to outline a basic course in industrial nursing for colleges and universities. Content included the role and functions of the industrial nurse, set-up of the medical department, scope of industrial nursing services, the nurse's role in health education, collaborative relationships of the industrial nurse, standing orders, record-keeping, legal aspects of industrial nursing, production factors, accidents and medical problems, and trends in industrial health (AAIN, 1944).

From 1945 to 1947, Fortune (1947) conducted a survey of 32 baccalaureate nursing programs. One of the purposes was to examine industrial nursing course content within these programs. Findings indicated that 13 of the schools offered one or more isolated courses in industrial nursing. Most of the faculty teaching these courses had limited, if any, industrial nursing exposure.

Education in industrial nursing in the 1950s continued to evolve. The Smith (1952) study at Yale University revealed that the nursing school curriculum had been enriched with socioeconomic and health issues relevant to occupational health, but many concepts about industrial or occupational health nursing practice and related fields of knowledge were lacking. There was continued need for faculty reevaluation and course content revision.

At the 1958 American Nurses' Association convention, the Industrial Nursing Section voted to change the name industrial nursing to occupational health nursing (The 1958 Convention, 1958). About the same time a major curriculum study (Henriksen, 1959), funded by a grant from the *American Journal of Nursing* to the Minnesota League for Nursing, was conducted to determine the essentials of occupational health that should be included in the basic collegiate nursing program. Separately developed questionnaires were sent to all known occupational health nurses ($N = 225$) and to 116 employers in Minnesota. The investigator sought to identify important functions specific to the field of occupational health nursing and to delineate trends in occupational health programs as the basis for educational preparation. Eighty percent of occupational health nurses and 70% of employers completed the questionnaire. A high degree of agreement regarding activities and trends was demonstrated by both groups. In addition, nursing curricula in six Minnesota collegiate schools of nursing were examined in terms of occupational health content.

Most occupational health nurses were diploma school graduates and much of their learning was by trial and error. Nursing school curricula did not emphasize the occupational health component, even when health problems had occupational implications. Management was unaware of the knowledge and skills needed by occupational health nurses. Recommendations from the project included strengthening nursing school curricula within specific occupational health courses, integrating occupational health nursing concepts into basic curricula, and informing management about the qualifications needed for occupational health nurses (Henriksen, 1959).

In 1964 another study was conducted to test the hypothesis that content necessary to prepare occupational health nurses was included in baccalaureate programs. Two schools participated in the study, Boston University and the University of Tennessee. In the Boston project a checklist of 18 major subject areas was developed and used by the faculty to assess curriculum content. Only 44% of the items on the checklist were included in the curriculum (Summers, 1967). Concluding after 1 year, the Boston University project results indicated that there was some occupational health nursing content in the school curriculum but the content area needed strengthening.

The University of Tennessee project (Keller, 1970) lasted 4 years. Initially, occupational health nursing competencies and content for practice were identified. As the competencies emerged, relevant academic content in occupational health was identified for each competency and was stated at the expert level of professional nursing in occupational health. Course content included in the curriculum was then described by faculty, and observations of content by the same investigator through class auditing experiences were used for validation. The researcher concluded that occupational health nursing content should be integrated much more throughout the curriculum with emphasis on prevention, health promotion, and developing and utilizing a conceptual or theoretical model.

Brown (1976) conducted a study of 40 randomly selected NLN accredited baccalaureate nursing programs to determine if specific occupational health nursing content related to effects of work on health, influence of health on work, occupational health legislation, and occupational health program management were included in the curricula. The results indicated that 56% of the 27 responding schools had content in all four areas, with 70% of the content taught in community health nursing courses. Field experience seldom was offered.

To support further the importance of education in occupational health nursing, the American Association of Occupational Health Nurses surveyed a random sample of the membership (Cox, 1983), and 49% responded that company management suggested and encouraged participation in both academic and continuing education. In addition, 90% of companies compensated for educational programs.

In 1986 Rogers surveyed all NLN accredited baccalaureate programs in the United States ($N = 425$) to examine the inclusion of eight major content areas and 53 subcontent areas within curricula. Major content areas included environmental health nursing, environmental health issues, occupational and environmental legislation, basic occupational health nursing concepts, occupational health nursing practice, effects of work on worker health, management concepts, and related fields of knowledge (e.g., industrial hygiene, epidemiology, toxicology). Of the 222 (53%) schools responding, 215 (51%) reported having some content in occupational health nursing. However, major content areas specifically related to occupational health nursing concepts and practice, related fields of knowledge, and management of the occupational health unit were reported as included in the curriculum by less than 50% of the respondents. Occupational health nursing faculty or guest lecturers taught less than 10% of the time, with community health nursing faculty responsible for the bulk of the teaching. Thirty percent of respondents reported that students were provided a field or observational experience. As 47% of schools did not respond to the survey, one should question if nonresponse indicated lack of occupational or environmental health content in the curriculum (Rogers, 1991).

Using a modification of the tool developed by Rogers (1991), Chitnis (1987) examined the opinions of practicing occupational health nurses regarding inclusion of occupational and environmental health nursing content in baccalaureate programs. These opinions were compared with curricular content as reported by nursing educators in Rogers' study. More than three-fourths of the practicing occupational health nurses recommended that all major content areas be included in baccalaureate nursing programs excepting the area of environmental health-related concerns; however, nearly 60% of occupational health nurses considered this area important to include in the curriculum.

Olson and Kochever (1989) examined occupational health and safety content in the curricula among baccalaureate schools of nursing in the Midwest. A self-administered questionnaire was mailed to 73 deans. On a scale of 1 (low) to 3 (high), respondents were asked to indicate the degree to which 27 occupational health and safety content areas were integrated into the curriculum. Fifty-two schools responded that health promotion, health education, worker's compensation and the Occupational Safety and Health Act were integrated most frequently.

Fewer studies or reports have been published regarding clinical occupational health nursing experiences. Miller and Skinner (1982) interviewed 54 junior nursing students and staff occupational health nurses after placing them in an occupational health setting for their community health clinical experience. Students were able to practice their skills in assessing and caring for workers and participated in individual and group health teaching. Students believed they were able to meet their objectives and gained a better understanding of the interrelationship of work and health.

A 10-week program in occupational health nursing was offered at St. Elizabeth Medical Center, Granite City, Illinois by nursing faculty members from Southern Illinois University in collaboration with the Industrial Medicine Program from St. Elizabeth's (Lepping, 1985). The program provided the opportunity to examine organizational structure, labor management, and the role of the occupational health nurse. Primary, secondary, and tertiary levels of prevention, toxicology, ergonomics, occupational diseases, assessment, observation, counseling, and health education skills were discussed and utilized. Students used the work area for their practice. Based on positive student and nurse evaluations, the occupational health concept was added to the baccalaureate curriculum at Southern Illinois University in Edwardsville.

This program exemplifies collaborative efforts involving occupational health nurses and educators.

Glugover (1985) reported successful utilization of an occupational health site for baccalaureate students at East Stroudsburg University in Pennsylvania. Ten industries were selected for clinical practice in community health nursing; in most places a nurse was not employed. Objectives were developed during the 15-week semester, and students were expected to assess health and safety hazards, preexisting programs for safety and wellness, and characteristics of the worker population. Students shared their experiences and ideas in the classroom. They were helped to recognize health needs and were involved in health screening, follow-up screening, health education, and wellness orientation. As a result of this program, students verbally reported in group sessions an increased understanding of nurse professionalism and the role and scope of practice in occupational health nursing. They also became more aware of occupational and environmental hazards, environmental protection, and health promotion issues in industries dealing with toxic waste products.

In another evaluation of student clinical experience (Prestholdt & Holt, 1989), pairs of 50 senior nursing students participated in a practicum experience in occupational health provided by a large southern university. Students were placed in three petrochemical occupational health departments for 18 hours per week for 3 weeks. Student objectives were developed to include the following:

- promote safety among groups of clients;
- reduce or eliminate accidental hazards in the workplace;
- examine principles of epidemiology applied to employee health;
- practice strategies appropriate for clients from a variety of cultural backgrounds;
- differentiate psychological and physiological growth and development patterns across the life span;
- refine modalities of client assessment;
- examine interpersonal intervention strategies related to client responses to stress.

Students' evaluations were consistently rated as excellent, particularly as to meeting the course objectives, developing increased independence in practice and learning more about community resources (Prestholdt & Holt, 1989).

SUMMARY

Since the early 1900s, several studies have been conducted to examine specifically content in nursing curricula related to occupational health nursing practice. Attention to conceptual modeling was limited. Designs were descriptive, generally survey, with a wide range in sample size and type. Results consistently indicated lack of standardized programs; sporadic occupational health content offered; lack of occupational health nursing concepts, particularly related to prevention, practice interventions, and management; inadequate information on related fields of knowledge (e.g., toxicology, epidemiology, industrial hygiene); and minimal, if any, clinical practicums in occupational health settings. Numerous variations in the curricular offerings were reported. Whether courses specific to occupational health nursing or content integrated throughout the curriculum provided a better approach to curricular experiences was not clear.

In order to increase the understanding of the relationship of work and health and to develop strategies aimed at reducing hazards in the work environment, more emphasis needs to be placed on integrating occupational health nursing concepts and related fields of knowledge into basic nursing education. Concepts specific to primary, secondary, and tertiary prevention should be emphasized through applied clinical experiences.

GRADUATE EDUCATION

In 1985 Rogers surveyed all known graduate occupational health nursing programs and found that they varied in length, terminal objectives, and curricular content. Most programs were supported by funding from the National Institute for Occupational Safety and Health (NIOSH). In addition to appropriate clinical/practitioner content depending on the program of study, core content in the curricula generally included coursework in occupational health nursing, medicine, epidemiology, statistics, toxicology, industrial hygiene, safety, administration, research, and public health policy issues. Student practicum experiences or internships varied considerably in terms of presence or absence, type, and length of the experience. Seven of 15 programs surveyed prepared nurse clinicians or practitioners, whereas eight prepared nurse managers or occupational health specialists. Twelve of the programs admitted students on either a full- or part-time option; three admitted on a full-time basis only. Programs ranged in length from 4 quarters to 2 years and the terminal degree generally was master's. Since that time, four of these programs have offered a doctoral degree in occupational health nursing.

Lusk, Disch, and Barkauskas (1988) surveyed 400 American Association of Occupational Health Nurses members in the Midwest region (catchment area Michigan, Ohio, and Indiana) to determine interest, employer support, and barriers to entering academic programs. A total of 204 (51%)

questionnaires were returned. Most respondents (82%) believed that a master's degree in occupational health nursing was needed. Respondents reported that 40% of employers offered full tuition, and 37% offered partial tuition reimbursement. Barriers to advanced education most frequently cited were the need to maintain an income (64%), the need to maintain fringe benefits (58%), and the travel distance to the program (56%).

An analysis of employment patterns of master's-prepared occupational health nurses was done by McGovern and colleagues in 1985. A self-administered questionnaire was sent to 121 graduates of occupational health nursing programs, 73 (65%) responded. Questions were related to employer characteristics, job roles and functions, educational preparation, and perceived continuing education needs. All but two of the respondents were female, with a mean age of 37. Most respondents ($n = 39$) were employed in administrative roles, and the remainder worked as educators, practitioners, or in clinical roles. Major responsibilities were reported as education (38%), management (30%), direct care (30%), consultation (29%), and program development (24%). Most of the respondents worked in private industry (52%) or were employed in government facilities (35%). Most respondents believed they needed continuing education in computer applications, program planning and evaluation, management, and insurance risk management (Christensen, Richard, Froberg, McGovern, & Abanobi, 1985; McGovern, Richard, Christensen, Froberg, & Abanobi, 1985).

SUMMARY

Graduate programs in occupational health nursing have prepared nurses for advanced clinical or administrative positions and as educators and researchers. However, only a small number of nurses have been prepared at the master's level, and only a few are prepared with doctoral degrees in occupational health nursing. It is imperative that occupational health nurses with advanced skills be prepared to function in management and policymaking positions. Particularly, nurse researchers are needed to expand the knowledge base and field of study in occupational health nursing.

TRENDS AND FUTURE RESEARCH

In the United States baccalaureate education has included only a modest amount of occupational health nursing content. However, because of the increased recognition of the impact of work and the work environment on health in recent years, more interest in and emphasis on occupational health nursing content is being demonstrated (Olson & Kochevar, 1989). Also, the role of the occupational health nurse as a manager of health services has become increasingly evident and important in program cost-effectiveness (Rogers, 1990).

Graduate education is more available; however, the majority of nurses currently employed in occupational health settings are prepared at the diploma or associate degree level and would need baccalaureate degrees in order to enter graduate programs. Anecdotal conversations with practicing occupational health nurses indicate that they would prefer to complete a baccalaureate degree in which at least some emphasis is placed on occupational health nursing; however, this often is not available.

Almost all of the occupational health nursing content has reportedly been taught by community health nursing faculty rather than faculty prepared or practicing as occupational health nurses. This is due largely to the lack of prepared faculty in occupational health nursing; however, courses probably could be enhanced by participation of practicing occupational health nurses and collaboration with other disciplines in teaching related concepts. It is imperative that nurses be prepared at the doctoral level to conduct occupational health nursing research and to guide students' research. This needs to be a strong component of the curriculum.

Practicum experiences in occupational health settings seemed to be a valuable component and learning experience for the students. To work individually with employees to apply an aggregate-focused care has proven effective practice for students. However, all of the studies report minimal use of occupational health sites for either clinical or management practica. This type of experience should be developed and utilized further.

Future researchers should focus particularly on conceptualization of the field of occupational-health nursing. Existing frameworks for occupational health nursing practice and other related frameworks could be used by investigators to further develop the organization of knowledge in occupational health nursing.

Research on occupational health nursing education has been aimed primarily at the undergraduate level. However, many of these studies were hampered by methodological weaknesses so that a total picture of the scope of curricular content, particularly practicum experiences, is lacking. Many of the reports of practicum experiences were evaluations aimed more specifically at examining the fit of the experience or adequacy in meeting course objectives. Although these types of reports have been valuable, more sophisticated evaluation research could lead to a higher level of knowledge that could be applied to improve the learning experience.

Research on graduate education in occupational health nursing is sorely needed. Only three reports in the literature addressed differing topical areas in occupational health nursing, that is, types of programs, barriers to education, and employment characteristics (Lusk, 1988; McGovern, 1985; Rogers, 1985). No reports were found in which investigators carefully examined curricular content in graduate education, practicum experiences, faculty preparation, or research output of students. One explanation for this is that graduate programs in occupational health nursing have had a variable history. Only since the establishment of the National Institute for Occupational Safety and Health funded Educational Resource Centers (ERCs) in 1977 has there been a major effort to provide continuous graduate level occupational health nursing education. There currently are 14 ERCs in the United States, 12 of which have NIOSH approved occupational health nursing graduate programs either in schools of nursing or public health.

Graduate education at the master's level prepares individuals for administrative, occupational health specialist, or advanced clinical positions; most programs are usually 1 to 2 years in length. Program accessibility and flexible options need careful consideration as more and more students are electing part-time study. In addition, more nurses without occupational health nursing backgrounds are entering the field. This will impact on curricular modeling, and careful monitoring of curricula programming is needed to ensure current and appropriate content. Current models may need to vary to some extent depending on the terminal product produced such as practitioner, manager, or occupational health specialist. Suboptions such as hospital employee health, nursing in highly technological settings, and nursing in space must be considered when planning and revitalizing nursing curricula (Rogers, 1990).

Research on innovations in educational programs has not been reported. For example, alternative practicum experiences at the undergraduate and, particularly, graduate level need to be examined to determine the best possible learning situation. This would include a comparison of types of preceptors necessary to provide needed mentorship.

In addition, evidence is needed that curricula are meeting the needs of occupational health nurses in occupational health settings. Considerable research needs to focus on outcomes of graduate education related to types of jobs, job satisfaction, congruence with educational preparation, and research productivity. Documentation is needed on the effectiveness of the master's-prepared occupational health nurse in employment settings.

REFERENCES

The 1958 Convention. (1958). *American Journal of Nursing, 58*, 7.
American Association of Industrial Nurses. (1944). *Outline of basic college course for industrial nurses.* Unpublished paper. New York: Author.

American Association of Occupational Health Nurses. (1988). *Standards of occupational health nursing practice*. Atlanta: Author.

Brown, E. M. (1976). Summary of a descriptive study of the occupational health nursing content in baccalaureate curricula of selected schools of nursing. *Occupational Health Nursing, 24*, 9–12.

Chitnis, S. (1987). *A descriptive study of occupational health nurses' views on including occupational and environmental health content in baccalaureate nursing curricula*. Unpublished master's thesis. Chapel Hill, NC: University of North Carolina.

Christensen, M., Richard, E., Froberg, D., McGovern, P., & Abanobi, O. (1985). An analysis of the employment patterns, roles and functions of master's prepared occupational health nurses—Part II. *Occupational Health Nursing, 33*, 453–459.

Cox, A. (1983). AAOHN education survey. *Occupational Health Nursing, 31*, 28.

Fortune, E. (1947). A comparative study of the content of courses and programs in industrial nursing with the duties of nurses employed in industry. Unpublished manuscript. Washington, DC: The Catholic University of America.

Glugover, D. (1985). Community health nursing students working and learning in the workplace. *Occupational Health Nursing, 33*, 286–288.

Henriksen, M. (1959). *Curriculum study of the occupational health aspects of nursing—An adventure in cooperation*. Minneapolis, MN: University of Minnesota.

Keller, M. (1970). *Occupational health content in baccalaureate nursing education*. Washington, DC: U.S. Government Printing Office.

Lepping, G. (1985). Mentorship in occupational health nursing. *Occupational Health Nursing, 33*, 547–549.

Lusk, S., Disch, J., & Barkauskas, V. (1988). Barriers to advanced education for occupational health nurses. *AAOHN Journal, 36*, 457–463.

Miller, P., & Skinner, S. (1982). Use of occupational health setting for nursing student experiences. *Occupational Health Nursing, 30*, 31–33.

McGovern, P., Richard, E., Christensen, M., Froberg, D., & Abanobi, O. (1985). An analysis of the employment patterns, roles and functions of master's prepared occupational health nurses—Part I. *Occupational Health Nursing, 33*, 407–413.

McGrath, B. (1946). *Nursing in commerce and industry*. New York: The Commonwealth Fund.

National Organization for Public Health Nursing. (1941). A study of industrial nursing services. *Public Health Nurse, 33*, 219–224.

Olson, D., & Kochevar, L. (1989). Occupational health and safety content in baccalaureate nursing programs. *AAOHN Journal, 37*, 33–38.

Prestholdt, C., & Holt, B. (1989). Enhancing baccalaureate student nursing education: Collaboration with occupational health nurses for hands-on-experience. *AAOHN Journal, 37*, 465–469.

Rogers, B. (1985). Graduate education in occupational health nursing. *Occupational Health Nursing, 33*, 204–205.

Rogers, B. (1990). Occupational health nursing practice, education and research: Challenges for the future. *AAOHN Journal, 38*, 536–543.

Rogers, B. (1991). Occupational health nursing education: Curricular content in baccalaureate programs. *AAOHN Journal 39*, 101–108.

Smith, E. (1952). *Occupational health integration in the Yale School of Nursing* (League Exchange No. 1). New York: National League for Nursing.

Summers, V. (1967). An occupational health nursing study. *Nursing Outlook, 15,* 64–66.

Whitlock, O. M., Tasko, M. V., & Kohl, F. R. (1944). *Nursing practices in industry* (Public Health Bulletin 283). Washington, DC: U.S. Government Printing Office.

PART IV

Research on the Profession of Nursing

Chapter 9

Mentorship

Connie Nicodemus Vance
School of Nursing
The College of New Rochelle

Roberta Knickrehm Olson
School of Nursing
The University of Kansas

CONTENTS

The concept of mentorship in the nursing profession has attracted growing interest, particularly within the last decade. Role socialization, including career development, is a continuous developmental process proceeding through specific life stages from childhood through adulthood. It is now recognized that the presence of a mentor is crucial to the role socialization and career development of the professional person. The classic mentor–protégé relationship is one in which an older, more experienced person guides, supports, and nurtures a younger, less experienced one. Levinson, Darrow, Klein, Levinson, and McKee (1978) view the mentor as both "parent" and "older peer," whose efforts and special concern push the protégé toward realizing full potential. The mentoring relationship consists of a variety of roles and behaviors that contribute to both the personal and professional development of the protégé. Like a role model, the mentor demonstrates desired behaviors, thus enhancing the learning experience. In addition to being a role model, however, the mentor personalizes the modeling influences by becoming involved directly with the protégé in a continuing relationship. A mentor may serve, therefore, as a role model, guide, teacher, tutor, coach, confidant, and visionary-idealist (Vance, 1982).

The complexity of nursing practice requires an ongoing support system for both new as well as advanced practitioners. Mentor–protégé relationships can provide various types of socialization and support to all levels of nursing professionals at various points in their careers. Nurse researchers have begun to investigate mentorship within the profession. A line of research as well as a growing body of literature related to the nature, benefits, and outcomes of mentoring for nurses has emerged.

There have been several excellent literature reviews of the mentoring process in various fields, including nursing (Bolton, 1980; Hall & Sandler, 1983; Jowers & Herr, 1990; Merriam, 1983; Moore, 1982). The doctoral study completed by Vance in 1977 was the first study to define and investigate systematically the mentor concept in the nursing profession. Therefore, 1977 was selected as the beginning period for tracing mentorship research for the present review, which is focused on mentorship research in the nursing field for a 14-year period (1977–1990). Because investigation of the concept of mentoring, as specifically applied to nursing, has been a recent development, a variety of methods were employed to locate the studies for this review.

Manual and computer searches were conducted to identify master's postmaster's, doctoral, postdoctoral, faculty, and nursing service research. *Master's Abstracts International* (MAI) and *Dissertation Abstracts International* (DAI) were important sources, as well as the *Cumulative Index to Nursing and Allied Health Literature*. A letter was sent to the heads of National League for Nursing accredited masters and doctoral programs in the United States ($N = 140$) and Canada ($N = 12$), explaining the purpose of the project and soliciting names of faculty and students in the school, or other nurses, who were conducting mentor research.

A letter was sent to the editors of 10 journals in the United States and Canada, asking them to publish a *Call for Information* about published or unpublished studies in the area of mentorship. The journals selected were: *Research in Nursing and Health, Nursing Outlook, Nurse Educator, Journal of Nursing Administration, Nursing Research, Image: Journal of Nursing Scholarship, Journal of Nursing Education, Nursing Administration Quarterly, The Canadian Nurse,* and *Nursing Papers* (Canada). The majority of journals complied with the request. The establishment of personal contacts occurred through our consultation and presentation activity, thesis and dissertation committee service, as well as attendance at conferences and conventions, including the First International Conference on Mentoring in Vancouver, British Columbia, in 1986.

Through this extensive search process, 54 studies on mentoring in nursing have been located. Criteria for inclusion in this review were: (a) research-based; (b) related to the nursing profession; and (c) conducted between 1977–1990. Because this is a developing line of research in nursing (just a little over a decade old), there are only a few published studies. Therefore, the majority of studies reviewed are doctoral or master's investigations. Given the current status of the research, this is still pioneering, mostly unpublished, exploratory work.

The studies in this review are presented in seven categories under the major heading of *Mentor Relationships for Career Development:* (a) mentoring of baccalaureate students, (b) mentoring of new graduates, (c) mentoring of staff nurses, (d) mentoring of graduate students, (e) mentoring among nurse educators, (f) mentoring among academic and service administrators, and (g) mentoring among nurse-influentials. From our review, it is apparent that mentoring is occurring at all levels of educational preparation in the nursing profession and at various stages of the nursing career. The majority of reported studies, however, occur at leadership levels or advanced career stages.

NATURE OF THE MENTOR RELATIONSHIP

Mentoring is a concept that presents complex definitional and methodological issues for researchers (Carmin, 1988; Fagan, 1988). Many variables affect the nature of the mentor–protégé relationship such as sex, age, and experience of the participants; the level of intensity and length of the relationship; stage of the career of both mentor and protégé; and the types of roles and functions that both the mentor and protégé bring to the relationship. Erikson's work (1963, 1968) has provided an important theoretical foundation for viewing mentoring as part of the developmental process termed "generativity," in which the primary concern is establishing and guiding the next generation.

Bandura's (1977) social learning theory provides another theoretical foundation for mentoring. This theory is based on imitation of modeling behavior of another. The value of learning through modeling, as compared to trial and error learning from consequences of one's actions, is to acquire a larger, better integrated behavior pattern more quickly.

MENTOR RELATIONSHIPS FOR CAREER DEVELOPMENT

Authors interested in the concepts of vocational life stages and career development suggested that some form of mentoring relationship is important at each stage of a professional person's career (Dalton, Thompson, & Price, 1977; Hall, 1976). Using Super's (1957) model of vocational life stages, Vance (1977, 1986) developed prototypes of mentoring influences that were important in the careers of the nurse influentials she investigated. This paradigm of mentor types included the parent–sponsor, intellectual–guide, sociocultural role model, visionary–idealist, promoter–coach, peer–colleague, and mentor emeritus. The present review illustrates the nature of the mentor relationship in the nursing profession at all stages of a nursing career—from early to advanced.

Mentoring of Baccalaureate Students

Chappell (1983), Dimino (1986), and Gresley (1986) conducted studies of senior students in baccalaureate programs. Chappell (1983) described the role and responsibilities of the preceptor during the students' senior-year experience. Through literature review and structured interviews, a model of mentoring concepts was developed for both student and preceptor. Dimino (1986) studied 12 senior nursing students and their preceptor-mentors in a perioperative nursing elective in a university program. The purpose of the study was to increase student knowledge and skill in providing perioperative nursing care to children and to ease the students' transition to professional nursing practice. The students reported that the mentoring experience enhanced their communication, technical, and organizational skills and provided an opportunity to explore how a nursing career would influence their quality of life. The staff preceptors reported this experience as rewarding; in addition, it provided an opportunity to enhance their teaching skills. Gresley (1986) studied 34 senior students and their mentors in the last quarter of their baccalaureate nursing program. Pre- and post-test data from the Tennessee Self-Concept Scale (Fitts, 1965) and the Six-Dimensional Scale of Nursing Performance (Schwirian, 1977, 1979) revealed significant gains in student scores as analyzed with a t-test.

The reciprocal benefits of mentoring are illustrated in these three studies. Although the samples were small, the researchers reported that mentorship programs assist students in skill development and self-confidence and enhance preceptor-mentors' teaching skills and stimulate their learning.

Mentoring of New Graduates

Transition into the role of nurse as a new graduate has been studied by Atwood (1979, 1981), Smith (1985), Shields (1986), Murray (1987), and Hamilton, Murray, Lindholm, & Myers (1989). The transitional process of 10 new graduates to a hospital work setting was analyzed by Atwood (1979, 1981), using the Performance Expectations for New Graduate Nurses (Benner, Colavecchio, Field, & Gordon, 1980) and the Klahn Self-Concept Scale (Ward & Fetter, 1979), along with anecdotal records and mentee diaries. The self-concept of the new graduate was high on the pre-test and reflected the security of recent classroom theory. The mentors' self-concept scores were lower than the mentees', but the changes in the mentors' pre- and post-test scores were significantly greater than the mentees' and reflected the stimulus and renewal created by participation in the program. All of the mentors, without exception, indicated a greater awareness and understanding of themselves following this experience.

Smith (1985) investigated mentoring outcomes for the protégé, the mentor, and the organization in a critical-care setting following a formalized mentoring nurse intern program. No significant differences were found for interns ($n = 42$) and noninterns ($n = 55$) in educational achievement, professional identity, and extended job responsibilities as measured by a researcher-developed, registered nurse, career-development questionnaire. The mentor outcome was examined by comparing responses between 24 head-nurse mentors to a standard measure of professional burnout on three variables: emotional exhaustion, depersonalization, and personal accomplishment. No significant difference in responses was found except for the head-nurse mentors' greater intensity of emotional exhaustion and greater frequency and intensity on depersonalization items. The investigator stressed the need for additional research to evaluate the relationship of mentoring to the nursing profession. The Kentucky Mentoring Survey (Fagan & Fagan, 1982) was used by Shields (1986) to describe the mentoring relationships reported by 126 clinical nurses on entering the profession. The majority of nurses experienced mentoring relationships that were perceived as facilitating their career development. The mentors were, in general, senior colleagues of the same sex and race who taught technical aspects and role modeled desirable professional characteristics. As they became "experienced" nurses, the protégés subsequently assumed a mentoring relationship with new graduates.

Murray (1987) evaluated the differences between a group of orientees with baccalaureate-prepared preceptors ($n = 6$) and a group of orientees with nonbaccalaureate preceptors ($n = 9$) in one hospital setting, using the Six-Dimensional Scale by Schwirian (1979). Using a t-test, baccalaureate-prepared preceptors were evaluated as significantly more effective than non-baccalaureate preceptors in the areas of teaching and collaboration. The investigator suggested expanding the study to additional hospital settings to determine if the educational level should be a significant criterion in selecting preceptors for new staff nurse orientation.

Hamilton et al. (1989) conducted a quasi-experimental study for the purpose of determining how mentors would affect the role transition and retention of new graduates. The seven experimental group subjects were assigned to one unit with the mentor with whom they worked for 3 months available on each shift. The 16 control-group subjects were assigned to various units. Each had a mentor, but the mentor did not work the same shift consistently as the protégé. Data were collected with the Minnesota Satisfaction Questionnaire (MSQ) (Weiss, Davis, England, & Lofquist, 1967) and the Leader Behavior Description Questionnaire (LBDQ) (Stogdill, 1963). Job satisfaction and perceived leadership behaviors revealed significant differences for those who were in the experimental group and mentored for three months. Consistent feedback regarding the integration of skill acquisition along with expected behaviors of the new graduate were seen as benefits from being mentored over time.

The investigators in these studies did not differentiate between the concepts of preceptor and mentor. The descriptive nature and small sample size of the studies limits their generalizability. The mutual benefits to both the protégé (i.e., new graduate) and the mentor were stressed, as well as the important role that mentors or preceptors play in the successful transition of the new graduate to that of clinician. The refinement of outcome measures, which is still a very exploratory area of research, as well as replication studies would provide a greater confidence level in supporting the findings related to outcomes of the mentoring process.

Mentoring of Staff Nurses

The next career phase to be described is "more experienced" staff nursing. Pyles and Stern (1983; Pyles, 1981), Fagan and Fagan (1982), Johantgen (1985), Hauser (1986), Hinson (1986), and Just (1989) studied staff nurses along the career continuum.

Pyles (1981, 1983) explored the phenomenon of neophyte nurses as they learned the role of the critical care nurse. Data were gathered from interactions and in-depth interviews with 28 registered nurses to determine the cognitive processes used in the development and application of assessment and decision-making skills in the early detection of cardiogenic shock in patients with myocardial infarction. The qualitative data indicated that the nurses with mentors used less trial-and-error methodology and arrived at the nursing diagnosis faster, more accurately, and with increased confidence in their abilities as a nurse.

Fagan and Fagan (1982) studied mentorship experiences for nurses ($n = 87$), police officers ($n = 70$), and public school teachers ($n = 107$). Nurses and teachers reported more mentor relationships than did police officers. Data from the nurses revealed a high correlation between being mentored and job satisfaction. Staff nurses who had been in practice more than 2, but less than 6 years were surveyed by Johantgen (1985) in order to identify the prevalence of mentor relationships and their effect on early career satisfaction and career development. The 121 nurse respondents reported that mentor relationships early in their career were very important. Many nurses noted that having several helping relationships was preferable to having only one. Even though mentor relationships were considered desirable, no significant differences were found in the mentored and nonmentored groups with regard to career satisfaction, career advancement, or tendency to be mentors to others.

Hauser (1986) interviewed 8 nurses for the purpose of investigating their perceptions of guiding-supporting relationships that exist in clinical practice settings. Analysis of the interview data revealed that a variety of persons served as their mentors. Major outcomes of these guiding-supporting relationships were career development, improved problem-solving abilities, and enhanced self-esteem. Seven major categories evolved to describe the processes by which these outcomes were achieved: sharing information and skills, encouraging, advising, role-modeling, providing feedback, providing logistical support, and caring. Hinson (1986) attempted to determine if staff nurses have mentors who assist in their career development. Major findings indicated that staff nurses in the study had mentors who contributed to their career development and that nurses both benefit from having mentors and being a mentor.

The frequency and nature of mentor relationships among staff nurses employed in acute care hospitals as well as the relationship betwen presence of a mentor and nurses' professionalism was investigated by Just (1989). A convenience sample of 157 full-time, female registered nurses who had worked at least one year as staff nurses completed the Mentor Survey, the Nurses' Self-Description Form (Dagenais & Meleis, 1982) and a Biographical Data Inventory. The Mentor Survey and Biographical Data Inventory were developed by the researcher. A subscale of the Nurses' Self-Description Form was used as a measure of professionalism. A significant difference was found between the mean professionalism scores of mentored and nonmentored nurses, with mentored nurses achieving higher scores. Responses indicated that a majority (73%) of the sample staff nurses engaged in mentor relationships. Most of these nurses identified two or more mentors in their lives, who were likely to be older staff nurses and who were acquired during the first year of employment. The mentoring relationships lasted an average of 2½ years.

These studies of staff nurses revealed that the presence of mentors enhanced problem-solving and decision-making, assisted in career guidance and support, and increased self-confidence. It was reported that more than one person and a variety of types of persons served as mentors. In-depth interviews appear to capture the process and the longitudinal developmental nature of the mentor phenomenon in contrast to the questionnaire-only format.

Mentoring of Graduate Students

Studies were conducted by Duane (1986) and Sealy (1987) with master's students. Zimmerman (1983), Young (1985), and Andersen (1986) studied doctoral students.

Master's Students.   Duane (1986) studied 41 master's students in the nursing administration major at one university. The questionnaire developed by Spengler (1982) was used to determine the characteristics and frequencies of mentor–protégé relationships in graduate students. Forty-six percent reported having a mentor; 54% reported two or more mentors. All of the respondents indicated that a mentor–protégé relationship was important in career development, but did not guarantee career planning or satisfaction. Duane stated that the value and outcomes of the mentor–protégé relationship should be addressed by the profession in order to assist the development of potential nurse leaders. A survey of 126 female Canadian master's nursing students was conducted by Sealy (1987) using a researcher-developed, mail questionnaire to explore perceptions of their mentor relationships. No significant differences were found between the demographic profiles of the nurses who had or had not experienced mentor relationships. The students wanted mentors to be supportive and inspirational and to provide assistance with the development of functional skills. The career assistance provided by mentors raised their levels of self-assurance and self-confidence and helped them feel "cared about" as they progressed toward achieving professional and personal goals.

Doctoral Students.   Zimmerman (1983) studied a random selection of 236 doctorally prepared female nurses in order to describe and examine the factors that most facilitated their career success. The Career Success Survey, developed by the researcher, served as the data-collection instrument. Personal characteristics were ranked as the most important factor in facilitating career success. The second-ranked factor facilitating career success was educational preparation; the third-ranked factor was significant others, or mentors. These mentors were identified as teacher, peer-colleague, and supervisor. They provided encouragement and recognition of potential, opportunities and responsibilities, and instruction and training. Young (1985) studied female doctoral students in nursing whose career goal was teaching and conducting research within a university setting. Major themes in critical incidents were collected through in-depth interviews. The critical incident focused on the student's initial mentor–protégé relationship and the perceived personal and career development related to that relationship. The protégé's perception of the conflict resolution process at different phases of the relationship was a crucial element in the ability to grow and develop from the relationship.

Andersen's (1986) phenomenological study examined the perceptions of 35 female doctoral students in nursing regarding their relationship with their dissertation committee chairpersons through an author-developed mail questionnaire and interview. The chairperson's power and influence was the most significant and the primary socializing agent for doctoral candidates. Relationships were more satisfying and productive when the chairperson was a role model, mentor, or sponsor who was experienced in the system, gave clear feedback and direction, and enhanced the student's self-esteem. Adverse relationships also were described.

The graduate nursing students (predominately female) in these studies testified to the significance of mentoring relationships as they proceeded with career development through advanced study. Caring, teaching, guidance, encouragement, and recognition of potential were identified as ingredients of a positive mentoring relationship. In a rare departure, one study examined sources of dissatisfaction in these relationships.

Mentoring Among Nurse Educators

Werley and Newcomb (1983), Olson (1984), Macey (1985), Vogt (1985), Hess (1986a), Jowers (1986), Kremgold-Barrett (1986), Tagg (1986), Williams (1986), and Wood (1990) have conducted studies of nurse educators in their first position and at various career points. Werley and Newcomb (1983) investigated the mentor concept and its potential for accelerating the development of nurse researchers as well as nursing research. A survey questionnaire developed by the researchers was mailed to the directors of the 21 current doctoral nursing programs to elicit information about explicit actions or behaviors from which mentor–protégé relationships might be inferred. Their findings suggested that interactional and structural factors do exist for faculty-student collaboration in research. However, there were relatively few collaborative publications based on joint research activity. The opportunity to work with a productive researcher was rated as a very important variable in developing a productive researcher. The authors advocated the growth of mentor–protégé relationships for the development of nurse researchers, and for advancing the growth of nursing research in the profession.

Olson (1984) studied the selection process of mentor–protégé relationships by 153 female nurse educators in college and university settings in 13 midwest states using mail questionnaires adapted from Vance (1977) and Spengler (1982). Data revealed that there was no signficant difference in career satisfaction whether a mentor–protégé relationship was assigned or selected. Structured interviews with 11 pairs of mentors and protégés revealed a trend toward greater career satisfaction when the relationship was selected mutually versus assigned. Responses from 275 full-time faculty in 32 NLN-accredited programs of nursing were analyzed by Macey (1985) regarding the existence of protégé–mentor relationships and whether they fostered faculty development. The author found that mentor relationships did exist, but did not increase faculty development (defined as involvement with publishing, research, professional organizations, university committees and community service). Faculty mentor relationships helped novice faculty to get into the system and become socialized to the sociopolitical climate of the school; they also provided the opportunity for the protégé to take on tasks formerly delegated to the mentor.

Vogt (1985) investigated the relationship of mentoring activity and career success of 144 nursing faculty from 5 randomly selected midwestern schools of nursing. Mentoring activity was measured with the Alleman's Leadership Development Questionnaire (1982). Although mentoring activity was reported, statistical analysis indicated no significant relationship between the total mentoring activity score and career success of nursing faculty. The findings indicated that programs on the mentoring process might improve the effectiveness of faculty mentoring in their organizations. Sixty-three nurse educators and 89 nursing service administrators were studied by Hess (1986a) to determine the frequency and characteristics of mentor–protégé relationships and whether these relationships affected career planning, career satisfaction or professional productivity. Differences between the two groups of subjects also were examined. Spengler's (1982) Mentor–Protégé Survey questionnaire was adapted to collect the information. Sixty percent of the respondents reported having a mentor. Mentoring did not appear to contribute a significant degree to career planning. The investigator concluded that mentoring is one method of facilitating career planning and development and that it enhances career satisfaction for potential nursing leaders.

Using mail-questionnaire data from 477 nurse female academicians, Jowers (1986) examined the mentor–protégé relationship with regard to the perceived degree of role conflict and role ambiguity. The survey included Mentor Scales (Pierce, 1983) and Role Ambiguity Index (Rizzo, House, & Lirtzman, 1970). There were significant inverse relationships between role ambiguity and all five of the variables that were studied: mentor behaviors, characteristics of the mentor relationship, power and achievement characteristics of the mentor, personal qualities of the mentor, and the protégés' achievements. Regression analyses revealed that the best predictors for a decrease in role ambiguity were characteristics of the mentor–protégé relationship, power and achievement characteristics of the mentor, and years at the present school.

A descriptive study conducted by Kremgold-Barrett (1986), explored mentoring relationships among women in a female-dominated environment though life stages and career development stages. Interviews were conducted with 15 faculty members from one university school of nursing. The investigator found that strong early role models served to demonstrate the importance and use of personal power, and that awareness of this power was crucial to later success in academia. In addition, feelings of collegiality, affirmation, and active mentoring were critical to assimilation into the faculty role and preparation for the tenure process. A sense of mastery and competence was important in attracting a support system. Additional findings were that administrative constraints sometimes inhibited mentoring and other supportive relationships.

In an effort to determine the existence of mentoring relationships among nurse faculty in the first 7 years of their career, Tagg (1986) conducted a retrospective study of 648 nurse faculty from 51 NLN-accredited baccalaureate programs. Faculty groups, with and without mentors, were compared. There was no significant diference between these two groups in relation to job satisfaction, burnout, rank, tenure, scholarly pursuits, or interest in being a mentor to others. The investigator concluded that many of the novice nurse educators lacked a mentor.

Williams (1986) and Williams and Blackburn (1988) focused on the relationship of mentoring by senior faculty to the productivity of junior faculty. Faculty from 8 of the top 20 schools of nursing ($N = 183$) responded to a mail questionnaire that was developed by Williams. Professionally stimulating environments contributed to the ability to predict research activity among junior faculty. Mentoring enhanced the productivity of senior faculty who were mentors. Book publishing and professional service, as measures of productivity, could be predicted by institutional and demographic variables of the sample. The study suggested that facilitation of a collaborative model for mentorship would increase the productivity of both junior and senior faculty.

A survey of 355 baccalaureate nursing faculty was carried out by Wood (1990) to determine the correlations among the faculty's teaching experience, the length of the faculty-supervisor relationship, and the supervisor's length of time in the role. The three top mentor roles used by supervisors in the study were demonstration of trust, teaching the job, and sponsoring the faculty member. The majority of faculty perceived the supervisor as a partial (51%) or full (15%) mentor. The supervisor had a high degree of influence on career (55%) and personal (43%) development. The overall relationship with the supervisor was positive, with the faculty reporting a high level of career satisfaction (71%).

In the preceding studies of academic nurses, the researchers investigated the relationship of mentoring to the development of scholarship; career planning, success, and satisfaction; and socialization into the faculty role. Statistically significant relationships were not found, for the most part, between mentoring and other variables; however, respondents frequently reported having a mentor/mentors. The mutual benefits of mentoring to both mentor and protégé were emphasized.

Mentoring Among Academic and Service Administrators

Academic Administrators. Academic deans were researched by Malone (1981), Bahr (1985), Alexander (1986), Fenske (1986), Schoolcraft (1986), White (1986, 1988), Castor (1987), and Rawl (1989). Malone (1981) studied the relationship of black female administrators' mentoring experience and career satisfaction. Administrators in university and business settings ($N = 130$) responded to the Career Experience Form, Minnesota Satisfaction Questionnaire (Weiss et al., 1967), and (Revised) Work Experiences Inventory. Forty-three of the subjects were nurses. A convenience sample of 6 mentored and 6 nonmentored administrators also were interviewed. No significant differences were found to support the research hypothesis that those administrators with a mentor relationship would report a higher level of career satisfaction. However, black female administrators who have multifaceted forms of professional support, including family, community, and a mentor relationship, reported greater satisfaction than those without multifaceted support.

The mentoring experiences of 10 women administrators in baccalaureate nursing education were described by Bahr (1985). They were asked in an interview to describe mentor relationships, career development, and advancement. Ninety percent of subjects who had a mentor perceived that they participated in a greater number of career development activities, completed a doctorate earlier, and moved into an administrative position sooner than did persons without a mentor. Alexander's (1986) study examined perceptions of the mentor relationship as it existed for 101 chief executive officers of NLN-accredited baccalaureate and higher degree nursing programs. Forty-two reported having a mentor and 59 did not have a mentor. Using the Adjective Check List (Gough, 1952), the participants were asked to describe factors that influenced the development of mentor–protégé relationships.

A study was conducted by Fenske (1986) of 43 male chief academic officers of education and 67 female chief academic officers of nursing. The purpose of the research was to compare the perceptions of mentoring relationships in the careers of the academic officers with regard to the characteristics and frequency of mentor–protégé relationships. A self-administered Mentoring Questionnaire, developed by the researcher, served for data collection. A majority of all the administrators had mentors. Comparison of data from the two groups revealed that: (a) females were appointed chief academic officers much sooner after earning doctoral degrees than were males; (b) most of the mentor–protégé relationships for the males occurred during the time that they were doctoral students and ended when they graduated or moved; most female mentor–protégé relationships ended when their mentors moved or died; (c) both males and females reported their willingness to serve as mentors; and (d) few subjects reported negative characteristics of mentor–protégé relationships.

Schoolcraft (1986) studied the relationship between mentoring and androgyny in 127 professors from three universities in the fields of business, education, and nursing. Data were collected with the researcher-developed Collegial Behaviors Inventory and the Bem Sex Role Inventory (Bem, 1981). The data revealed that there were no differences between: (a) men and women mentors in manifesting androgyny, (b) the three fields and the occurrence of sex-typed or androgynous sex roles, and (c) occurrence of sex-typed and androgynous sex roles among mentors. Significantly more nonmentors were sex-typed rather than androgynous.

Female academic nurse administrators were surveyed by White (1986, 1988) to determine their perceptions of the role of mentoring in career development and success. Three hundred chief academic officers in baccalaureate schools of nursing responded to a mail questionnaire developed by the researcher and indicated that they had a primary mentor, a secondary career mentor, or a significant individual in their lives who was considered important to their career development and success. White could not state that all academic nurse administrators need a mentor to succeed in their careers, but the majority of both mentored and nonmentored academic nurse administrators strongly supported the concept of mentoring for both career development and advancement.

Castor (1987) investigated facilitators, barriers, and alternatives to mentoring as perceived by nurse administrators of NLN-accredited baccalaureate nursing programs who indicated that they had had a protégé or a mentor. Structured interviews were conducted with 16 protégés and 9 mentors. Critical areas identified by both the mentor and the protégé in mentoring relationships were trust, personality characteristics, knowledge, interpersonal skills, and the environment. Alternatives to mentoring include relationships with significant others, collaborative professional activities, support groups, self-assessment, objective career planning, and development of a composite role model. Rawl (1989) studied variables related to career development for nursing education administrators. The 427 completed mail questionnaires (adapted from Olson, 1984) revealed that mentoring contributed significantly to the prediction of level of career development in becoming a nursing education administrator. Also important, however, was the individual's possession of an appropriate educational and experiential background.

Service Executives. Vice presidents for nursing, chief nurses, and head nurses have been examined for their mentoring relationships by Larson (1980, 1986), Taylor (1984), Knebel (1985), Giese (1986), Cardinali (1987), and Holloran (1989). Larson (1980, 1986) conducted an exploratory study of the differences in job satisfaction between nursing leaders in hospital settings who had a mentor and those who did not. Data were collected from 116 subjects with a questionnaire that contained the Job Descriptive Index (Smith et al., 1969) and items about characteristics of the respondents, including the presence or absense of a mentor relationship. Mentor relationships were present for the majority of the nursing leaders. Scores for those who had a mentor relationship were higher in the areas of satisfaction with work, promotion, supervision, and co-workers. Compared to those who were not mentors, respondents who were mentors to others had higher job satisfaction related to pay as well as the four areas just mentioned.

Giese (1986) replicated Larson's (1980) study with 64 nursing leaders in hospital settings. Findings supported the data analysis from Larson's study: (a) those who have mentors were more likely to be mentors; (b) satisfaction with work, supervisors and co-workers was higher in those who had mentors; and (c) satisfaction with work was higher in those who were mentors to others than those who were not. The data suggested that nursing administrators use mentor programs to socialize new nurse leaders in the hospital setting. Respondents from both studies perceived the need for management development for nurse leaders.

Taylor (1984) surveyed top nurse administrators in British Columbia about the type of mentoring help received. A researcher-developed mail questionnaire was returned by 119 subjects who were members of the Nurses Administrators' Association of British Columbia. Seventy-one percent of the respondents had one or more mentors. Mentored subjects indicated that they arrived at their present position through the encouragement and recommendation of another person or through taking advantage of unexpected job opportunities. Nonmentored respondents indicated that they arrived at their present position because they consistently worked toward this goal. More of the mentored subjects also served as mentors. Encouragement, recognition of potential, and inspiration to achieve high standards were rated as the most desirable kinds of mentoring help.

The role of the mentor relationship in the development of nurse leaders in hospital administrative positions was studied by Knebel (1985). Spengler's (1982) questionnaire was used to gather the data from 238 nurse leaders in one southern state. Fifty-seven percent of the respondents reported one or more mentor relationships. The mentor relationship was viewed positively by virtually all subjects and was characterized as intellectually stimulating, supportive, and growth-promoting. Competitiveness was identified by almost 50% of the subjects as the only negative chartacteristic.

Cardinali (1987) investigated the career development of 135 nurse executives in the United States Air Force Nurse Corps. Data from the mail questionnaire, adapted from Olson (1984), indicated that mentor relationships were not perceived as important to the subjects' own career development but were perceived as important in developing other nurses as administrators. Those who had mentor relationships mentored others. However, those relationships were not reported as important in job satisfaction.

Holloran (1989) studied the existence and nature of mentoring among female nursing service executives in medical center teaching hospitals. The self-report researcher-developed questionnaire, Mentoring in Nursing Service: A Survey of Nursing Service Executives, was completed by 274 respondents. Seventy-one percent had experienced a mentor relationship. The most beneficial aspect of the mentoring relationship was the encouragement and recognition of potential, inspiration and role modeling, the promotion of opportunities and responsibilities, and the demonstration of confidence in the protégé. A primary relationship was identified as having more impact than a secondary relationship on the career of the protégé. The primary mentor relationship included an emotional investment or commitment to the protégé's development.

Service Managers.   Hamilton (1984) investigated 65 nurse managers from 12 hospitals to determine if greater job satisfaction was experienced by managers who had a mentor relationship than by those who did not have a mentor. Differences in personal and career characteristics also were examined. Findings indicated a slight, but not statistically significant, difference in the job-satisfaction scores.

Differences in job satisfaction and role clarity between unit managers in hospital settings who had mentor relationships and those who had not were examined by Dunsmore (1987). Thirty-eight unit managers from 5 community hospitals responded to a questionnaire consisting of the Role Ambiguity Index (Rizzo et al., 1970), the Job Descriptive Index, (Smith et al., 1969), and career characteristics. Seventy-six percent reported a lack of formal training that was required for effective performance in their positions. Mentored managers reported significantly greater understanding of their role and greater satisfaction with opportunities for promotion.

Using the Leader Effectiveness and Adaptability Description (Hershey & Blanchard, 1982) with 26 head nurses, Hyland-Hill (1986) found no statistically significant differences between those who were mentored and those who were not. Head nurses who had a mentor were more likely to be mentor to others, and mentored subjects were younger than nonmentored subjects when they entered the role. A majority of the head nurses reported having a mentor.

The majority of administrators in these studies reported the presence of mentoring relationships, as mentor, protégé, or both. In general, findings indicated slight, but not statistically significant, relationships between being mentored and career satisfaction, development, and work advancement. Instrumentation is weak in this infant stage of investigation. Respondents strongly supported the mentor concept, perceived its importance in career enhancement, and were willing to serve as mentors. Two study investigators, Fenske (1986) and Schoolcraft (1986), compared male and female administrators' experiences in mentoring. One replication study (Giese, 1986) supported Larson's (1980) earlier findings related to mentor activity of nursing service administrators. Only one study reported negative characteristics of these relationships.

Mentoring Among Nurse Influentials

Nurse influentials are identified as leaders in nursing who have influenced the development of the profession. Researchers who have studied nurse influentials include Vance (1977, 1982), Spengler (1982), Lightfoot (1983), Hardy (1983, 1986), Larsen (1984), Kinsey (1985), and Slagle (1986).

Vance (1977, 1982) explored the structure of influence in the nursing profession. The names of nurse influentials were obtained by the reputational method, a nationwide nominating process. The 71 persons named most frequently were considered the nurse influentials and were included in the study. These individuals responded to a researcher-developed mail questionnaire that sought information on personal and family background, career characteristics, sources of influence and influence activities, and viewpoints of their profession. Data supported the research propositions that: influentials within the nursing profession would be situated in large urban settings; nurse influentials would report the presence of mentors in their lives; and both the positional leaders and the nurse influentials would agree on important sources of influence in nursing.

Kinsey (1985, 1986) conducted an updated group profile of contemporary nurse influentials and compared the data with the study by Vance (1977).

The comparison data included geographic locations, presence of mentors, and agreement on sources of influence. Forty-five nurse influentials identified by a nationwide nominating process completed a mail questionnaire and modified version of Flanagan's critical incident technique (1954). Data revealed that this group strongly resembled Vance's group in terms of their career characteristics. However, there was a substantial increase in academic-educational positions and publication and research activity among the current influentials. Academic pursuits and support systems were reported as the predominate critical factors associated with the nurse influentials' success. Career advice, guidance, and promotions were reported as the predominate favorable incident within a mentor relationship. Confrontation with mentors was the most frequently cited unfavorable incident.

Spengler (1982) explored the characteristics and frequency of the mentor–protégé relationships among female doctorally prepared nurses. The researcher-designed Mentor–Protégé Survey (MPS) was completed by 501 subjects. A majority (57%) had a mentor. Comparisons between mentored and nonmentored subjects revealed that those with mentors followed a definitive career plan more frequently, were more satisfied with their career progress, and had a greater sense of accomplishment related to career goals. No differences between the groups were noted with regard to research and scholarly activities.

Lightfoot (1983) explored the nature of mentoring relationships between eight mentor–protégé dyads of American Indian women within the nursing profession. Using the Vance (1977) methodology, these eight dyads responded to questions about personal and family background, professional and career characteristics, and mentoring activity. As a group, these nurses believed that their leadership development had been contingent on their own behavior or personal attributes, although a mentor relationship was considered to be a major influence on their development. The data suggested that both career and psychosocial assistance were part of the mentor relationship. A study by Hardy (1983, 1984) reported somewhat different findings from exploring the career histories of 35 leading female nurses in England and Scotland. Subjects were nominated by the reputational method used by Vance (1977), and data were gathered through mail questionnaires and interviews. Profiles revealed that most of the study subjects had spent a long period in their early careers without direction. The second career stage included establishment of a career and upward mobility. Mentoring relationships were an important factor for the study subjects in changing the tendency for lateral movement in the profession. In general, the respondents reported a high level of satisfaction with their nursing careers.

In an additional study, Hardy (1986) explored the career histories of selected leading male nurses in England and Scotland. The 13 male subjects were nominated to the study by the female nursing leaders studied by Hardy in

1983. Data were collected by a questionnaire and interviews. Two-thirds of the subjects reported having a mentor in their early career. Most of the subjects moved rapidly through a succession of positions after nursing school, with most subjects maintaining positions of influence that they had gained by their middle 30's. The study suggested that in contrast to the career patterns of female nurses, there are different expectations of men and women in nursing; these expectations may be working to the advantage of the male minority in the profession.

Based on interviews of 10 female, doctorally prepared professors in Canadian nursing schools, Larson (1984) concluded that career was a prominent, meaningful, and essential component of the subjects' adult lives. Mentoring relationships were not a common experience, whereas supportive female friends and colleagues were an ongoing aspect of their lives.

Twenty-five Fellows in the American Academy of Nursing who reside in the Northeast were interviewed by Slagle (1986) to determine elements inherent in mentoring relationships in their career development. Analysis of the interviews revealed that mentor–protégé relationships were a significant factor in their career development as leaders. The relationships were perceived as helpful and supportive, involving a mutual give-and-take process between the mentor and protégé that became more balanced as the relationship evolved. Relationships were affected by the protégés' abilities and needs, the career stage of the protégé, the talents and willingness of the mentor to help, and the setting of the relationship. The protégés usually became mentors to other nurses.

Exploration of the mentor concept with nurse influentials lends support to its presence and importance in career development and success. One replication study (Kinsey, 1985) updated a group profile of national nurse influentials and their career characteristics (Vance, 1977). In addition to the mail questionnaire and interviews, the researchers attempted to capture the complex nature of the relationship through case studies and autobiographical reports.

CONCLUSIONS AND RECOMMENDATIONS

For the most part the research on mentorship in nursing has been carried out within the last decade. The studies that were found consisted primarily of doctoral ($N = 33$) and master's ($N = 21$) studies, the majority of which are published in *Dissertation Abstracts International* or as unpublished master's theses. No studies were found in research journals. Several research reports were published in the following journals: *Image: Journal of Nursing Scholarship, Journal of Professional Nursing, Journal of Nursing Education, Journal of Nursing Staff Development, Nursing Administration Quarterly, Nursing and Health Care,* and *Nursing Outlook.* Three studies were reported in the *Proceedings of the First International Conference on Mentoring* (Gray & Gray, 1986).

The complex interactional, emotional, and longitudinal aspects of mentoring have made empirical measurement difficult. Carmin (1988) points out that this difficulty is complicated by a popular consensus of what mentoring is rather than from formal or operational definitions and subsequent empirical verification. The nursing studies in mentoring, as with those in other fields, are based on diverse definitions and theoretical formulations of the mentoring relationship. Nurse investigators have studied mentor relationships at various points in the nursing career (from the student phase through the advanced career stage) and in various milieu (academic, clinical, and administrative). Therefore, the theoretical framework and meaning of the concept frequently varied from study to study.

This review confirms the nature of the mentor relationship as process-oriented, developmental, and longitudinal. A combination of research methods, therefore, would be useful in examining these variables. Carmin (1988) suggested the employment of intensive representational case studies, observational methods, in-depth interviews, autobiographies, and diaries. Furthermore, she states: "With the greater accessibility and more widespread use of structural equations and causal modeling approaches, the study of such relationships has become more feasible and these techniques may provide a fruitful and innovative avenue of inquiry" (p. 11).

The researchers in these nursing studies used an exploratory or survey approach, which is appropriate, given the relative infancy of the topic. Self-report through questionnaires and interviews has been the major data-collection technique. Instrumentation has largely been researcher-developed, suggesting the need for validity and reliability testing of these instruments. The sample size of the studies is relatively small, and along with the descriptive nature of the studies, limits their generalizability.

Many of the researchers have attempted to validate the link between the mentoring phenomenon and career development, career success, and career satisfaction. The relationship between being mentored and mentoring others is also a common theme in the studies as well as the mutual benefits. Only a few researchers have attempted to document adverse aspects of the mentoring relationship. The exploratory results of this work are promising. However, with larger samples, more powerful instrumentation, use of comparison groups, and a longitudinal approach, greater confidence can be placed in the statistical significance of the findings. In addition, links may be validated between mentoring and other important variables to the nursing profession. McCloskey and Molen (1987) have indicated the importance of mentoring as a method of leadership development. The relationship of mentoring to adult growth and development is also in its nascent stages, and studies are needed to show how mentoring is related to adult development and adult learning (Merriam, 1983).

Two replication studies were found in this review: the Giese (1986) replication of the Larson (1980) study and the Kinsey (1985) replication of the Vance (1977) study. Replication will continue to be important in order to capture the longitudinal effects of the mentoring phenomenon as well as to confirm the validity and reliability of the findings and thereby add to this new line of investigation in mentorship.

Because many clinical and academic institutions are encouraging nurses and students to engage in mentoring activities through formal and planned mentoring programs, research is recommended in this area. Investigation of the structure, process, and outcomes of these programs will be necessary in order to encourage their development and expansion. These analyses may provide useful information about nonclassic definitions and new forms of the mentor system.

The nursing profession is predominantly female, and nursing studies in mentoring could yield greater insight into women's development, including both personal and professional arenas. Analysis and comparison of the female–female mentorship model with male–male or male–female models will provide important information to both the profession and to the women's studies area. There is still scant data regarding the dynamics of women mentoring women. Such investigations could include the characteristics of these relationships, for example the extent and varieties of mentoring influences and mentoring at career and personal transition points, and unique benefits and barriers to women mentoring women (Vance, 1986). Finally, the process of mentoring should be scrutinized more carefully, including the supports and barriers, the positive and the negative aspects, the reciprocal nature and the termination phases of these relationships.

It is clear that some type of support relationship is important in the career development, success, and satisfaction of professionals. Moreover, research in the area of mentoring has suggested that the mentoring relationship, as one form of support relationship, may be a crucial factor in building an effective and satisfying career. Further clarification of the mentoring phenomenon and its theoretical formulations as well as the refinement of the research methodology will assist in the understanding, initiation, and support of the mentor system in the nursing profession.

REFERENCES

Alexander, D. W. (1986). An investigation of deans' perceptions of attributes present in the mentor/mentee relationship (Doctoral dissertation, University of Texas at Austin). *Dissertation Abstracts International, 47,* 3703B.

Alleman, E. (1982). Mentoring relationships in organizations: Behaviors, personality characteristics, and interpersonal perceptions. (Doctoral dissertation, University of Akron). *Dissertation Abstracts International, 43,* 75A.

Andersen, S. L. (1986). The relationship between the doctoral student in nursing and her dissertation committee chairperson (Doctoral dissertation, Teachers College, Columbia University). *Dissertation Abstracts International, 47,* 1484B.

Atwood, A. H. (1979). The mentor in clinical practice. *Nursing Outlook, 27,* 714–717.

Atwood, A. H. (1981). Effects of a three-month mentorship on mentors and new graduate nurses in an acute care urban hospital (Doctoral dissertation, University of San Francisco). *Dissertation Abstracts International, 42,* 3817A.

Bahr, J. E. (1985). Mentoring experiences of women administrators in baccalaureate nursing education (Doctoral dissertation, Oklahoma State University). *Dissertation Abstracts International, 47,* 798A.

Bandura, A. (1977). *Social learning theory.* Englewood Cliffs, NJ: Prentice-Hall.

Bem, S. L. (1981). *Bem Sex-Role Inventory professional manual.* Palo Alto, CA: Counsulting Psychologist Press.

Benner, P., Colavecchio, R., Field, K., & Gordon, D. (1980). *Performance expectations of new graduate nurses.* San Francisco: AMICAE.

Bolton, E. B. (1980). A conceptual analysis of the mentor relationship in the career development of women. *Adult Education, 30,* 195–207.

Cardinali, M. A. (1987). *Mentoring relationships and career development among nurse administrators in the United States Air Force Nurse Corps.* Unpublished master's thesis, St. Louis University, St. Louis, MO.

Carmin, C. N. (1988). Issues in research on mentoring: Definitional and methodological. *International Journal of Mentoring, 2,* 9–13.

Castor, L. L. (1987). Mentoring: An analysis of facilitators, barriers, and alternatives. (Doctoral dissertation, The Pennsylvania State University). *Dissertation Abstracts International, 48,* 2549A.

Cearlock, H. (1986). *Nurses' involvement in marketing health services.* Unpublished master's thesis, Northern Illinois University, DeKalb.

Chappell, R. (1983). *The role of preceptor as an educational model in nursing at the baccalaureate level.* Unpublished master's project, South Dakota State University, Brookings.

Dalton, G. W., Thompson, P. H., & Price, R. L. (1977). The four stages of professional careers: A new look at performance by professionals. *Organizational Dynamics, 6,* 19–42.

Dagenais, F., & Meleis, A. (1982). Professionalism, work ethic, and empathy in nursing: The nurses self-description form. *Western Journal of Nursing Research, 4,* 407–422.

Dimino, E. (1986). *Senior BSN preceptorship in perioperative nursing.* Unpublished postmaster's study, Old Dominion University, Norfolk, VA.

Duane, S. J. (1986). *Mentor-protégé relationships: A study of career development among graduate nursing students.* Unpublished master's thesis, State University of New York, Buffalo.

Dunsmore, J. M. (1987). *A study to examine the differences in job satisfaction and role clarity of unit managers in hospital settings who have had mentor relationships and those who have not.* Unpublished master's thesis, University of Washington, Seattle.

Erikson, E. (1963). *Childhood and society.* New York: Norton.

Erikson, E. (1968). *Identity: Youth and crisis.* New York: Norton.

Fagan, M. M. (1988). The term mentor: A review of the literature and a pragmatic suggestion. *International Journal of Mentoring, 2,* 5–8.

Fagan, M. M., & Fagan, P. (1982). Mentoring among nurses. *Nursing and Health Care, 4,* 77–82.

Fenske, M. M. (1986). A comparison of the perceptions of mentoring relationships in the careers of female chief academic officers of nursing and male chief academic officers of education (Doctoral dissertation, George Peabody College, Vanderbilt University). *Dissertation Abstracts International, 47,* 2392A.

Fitts, W. (1965). *Manual for the Tennessee Self-Concept Scale.* Nashville, TN: Counselor Recordings and Tests.

Flanagan, J. (1954). The critical incident technique. *Psychological Bulletin, 51,* 328–357.

Giese, J. (1986). *A study to explore the differences in job satisfaction between nursing leaders in hospital settings who have had mentor relationships and those who have not.* Unpublished master's thesis, University of Washington, Seattle.

Gough, H. (1952). *Adjective checklist.* Palo Alto, CA: Consulting Psychologist Press.

Gray, W. A., & Gray, M. M. (Eds.). (1986). *Mentoring: Aid to excellence in career development, business, and the professions. Proceedings of the First Conference on Mentoring, II.* Vancouver, BC: International Association for Mentoring.

Greenwald, M. M. (1986). The nursing education executive position: Factors that influence leadership development (Doctoral dissertation, Teachers College, Columbia University). *Dissertation Abstracts International, 47,* 2371B.

Gresley, R. (1986). *The effects of mentorships in improving self-concept and professional role development in senior level baccalaureate nursing students.* Unpublished manuscript, Southern Illinois University, School of Nursing, Edwardsville.

Hall, D. T. (1976). *Careers in organizations.* Glenview, IL: Scott, Foresman.

Hall, R. M., & Sandler, B. R. (1983). Academic mentoring for women students and faculty: A new look at an old way to get ahead. *Project on the Status and Education of Women.* Washington, DC: Association of American Colleges.

Hamilton, E. M., Murray, M. K., Lindholm, L. H., & Myers, R. E. (1989). Effects of mentoring on job satisfaction, leadership behaviors, and job retention of new graduate nurses. *Journal of Nursing Staff Development, 5,* 159–165.

Hamilton, P. (1984). *An exploratory study of the relationship of a mentor on nurse manager job satisfaction.* Unpublished master's thesis, University of New Mexico, Albuquerque.

Hardy, L. K. (1983). *An exploration of the career histories of leading female nurses in England and Scotland.* Unpublished doctoral dissertation, University of Edinburgh, Scotland.

Hardy, L. K. (1984). The emergence of nursing leaders . . . a case of in-spite of, not because-of. *International Nursing Review, 31,* 11–15.

Hardy, L. K. (1986). *An exploration of the career histories of selected leading male nurses in England and Scotland.* Unpublished post doctoral study, University of Lethbridge, Lethbridge, Alberta, Canada.

Hauser, M. B. (1986). *Understanding guiding-supporting relationships in the clinical practice setting.* Unpublished master's thesis, Georgia State University, Atlanta.

Hershey, P., & Blanchard, K. W. (1982). *Management of organizational behavior: Utilizing human resources* (4th ed.). Englewood Cliffs, NJ: Prentice-Hall.

Hess, B. M. (1986a). *The role of mentors in the professional development of nurses: A comparative study.* Unpublished master's thesis, Washington State University, Seattle.

Hess, B. M. (1986b). The role of mentors in the professional development of nurses: A comparative study. In W. E. Gray & M. M. Gray (Eds.). *Proceedings on the First International Conference on Mentoring, II* (pp. 161–168). Vancouver, BC: International Association for Mentoring.

Hess, B. M. (1986c). Mentoring aids professional growth. *Washington Nurse, 16,* 21.

Hinson, D. K. (1986). Identification of the mentor relationship in the career of a staff nurse. (Master's thesis, University of Utah). *Master's Abstracts International, 25,* 199.

Holloran, S. D. (1989). Mentoring: The experience of nursing service executives. (Doctoral dissertation, Boston University). *Dissertation Abstracts International, 50,* 3920B.

Hyland-Hill, B. (1986). *Relationship between head nurse leadership effectiveness and presence or absence of a mentor.* Unpublished master's thesis, University of Washington, Seattle.

Johantgen, M. E. (1985). *The prevalence and effects of helping relationships on staff nurses' career development.* Unpublished master's thesis, State University of New York, Buffalo.

Jowers, L. (1986). Mentoring: Correlates with role conflict and role ambiguity of nurse academicians. (Doctoral dissertation, The University of Texas at Austin). *Dissertation Abstracts International, 47,* 1928–1929B.

Jowers, L., & Herr, K. (1990). A review of literature on mentor-protégé relationships. In G. Clayton and P. Baj (Eds.), *Review of Research in Nursing Education, III* (pp. 49–77). New York: National League for Nursing.

Just, G. (1989). Mentors and self-reports of professionalism in hospital staff nurses. (Doctoral dissertation, New York University). *Dissertation Abstracts International, 51,* 664B.

Kinsey, D. C. (1985). An updated group profile of contemporary influentials in American nursing. (Doctoral dissertation, Lehigh University). *Dissertation Abstracts International, 46,* 1870B.

Kinsey, D. C. (1986). The new nurse-influentials. *Nursing Outlook, 34,* 238–240.

Knebel, E. (1985). Profile of the mentor relationship in nursing service administration: A professional leadership development strategy. (Doctoral dissertation, University of Houston). *Dissertation Abstracts International, 46,* 3258A.

Kremgold-Barrett, A. (1986). Women mentoring women in academic nursing faculty. (Doctoral dissertation, Boston University.) *Dissertation Abstracts International, 46,* 588B.

Larsen, J. B. (1984). *A psychosocial study of the career development of selected nurses with earned doctoral degrees.* Unpublished doctoral dissertation, The University of Alberta, Edmonton, Canada.

Larson, B. A. (1980). *An exploratory study of the relationship of job satisfaction of nursing leaders in hospital settings who have had a mentor relationship and those who have not.* Unpublished master's thesis, University of Washington, Seattle.

Larson, B. A. (1986). Job satisfaction of nursing leaders with mentor relationships. *Nursing Administration Quarterly, 11*(1), 53–60.

Levinson, D., Darrow, C., Klein, E., Levinson, M., & McKee, B. (1978). *The seasons of a man's life.* New York: Ballantine.

Lightfoot, J. (1983). *An exploratory study of mentor relationships among American Indian women within the profession of nursing.* Unpublished master's thesis, The State University of New Jersey, Rutgers.

Macey, J. C. (1985). A study of faculty protégé-mentor relationships as a method for faculty development in schools of nursing. (Doctoral dissertation, George Peabody College, Vanderbilt University). *Dissertation Abstracts International, 46*, 1600A.

Malone, B. L. (1981). Relationship of black female administrators' mentoring experience and career satisfaction. (Doctoral dissertation, University of Cincinnati). *Dissertation Abstracts International, 43*, 558B.

Merriam, S. (1983). Mentors and protégés: A critical review of the literature. *Adult Education Quarterly, 33*, 161–173.

McCloskey, J. C., & Molen, M. T. (1987). Leadership in Nursing. In J. J. Fitzpatrick, & R. L. Taunton (Eds.). *Annual Review of Nursing Research, 5* (pp. 177–202). New York: Springer Publishing Co.

Moore, K. M. (1982). The role of mentors in developing leaders for academe. *Educational Record, 63*, 23–28.

Murray, R. C. (1987). *Effects of pairing a baccalaureate-prepared orientee with a preceptor of a generic baccalaureate program.* Unpublished post-baccalaureate study, Allentown College of St. Francis de Sales, Center Valley, PA.

Olson, R. (1984). An investigation of the selection process of mentor-protégé relationships among female nurse educators in college and university settings in the midwest. (Doctoral dissertation, St. Louis University). *Dissertation Abstracts International, 46*, 2259B.

Pierce, C. A. (1983). Mentoring, gender, and attainment: The professional development of academic psychologists. (Doctoral dissertation, The University of Texas, Austin). *Dissertation Abstracts International, 45*, 793A.

Pyles, S. H. (1981). *Assessments related to cardiogenic shock: Discovery of nursing gestalt.* Unpublished master's thesis, Northwestern State University of Louisiana, Shreveport.

Pyles, S. H., & Stern, P. N. (1983). Discovery of nursing gestalt in critical care nursing: The importance of the gray gorilla syndrome. *Image: Journal of Nursing Scholarship, 15*, 51–57.

Rawl, S. M. (1989). Nursing education administrators: Level of career development and mentoring. (Doctoral dissertation, University of Illinois, Chicago). *Dissertation Abstracts International, 50*, 1857B.

Rizzo, J. R., House, R. J., & Lirtzman, S. I. (1970). Role conflict and ambiguity in complex organizations. *Administration Science Quarterly, 15*, 150–163.

Rosenow, A. M. (1981). The dilemma of achievement in nursing: A woman's profession. (Doctoral dissertation, The University of Chicago). *Dissertation Abstracts International, 43*, 2311B.

Schoolcraft, V. L. (1986). The relationship between mentoring and androgyny. (Doctoral dissertation, The University of Oklahoma, Norman). *Dissertation Abstracts International, 47*, 3681A.

Schwirian, P. M. (1977). *Prediction of successful nursing performance* (Parts I and II, Publication No. HRA 77–17). Washington, DC: Department of Health, Education, and Welfare.

Schwirian, P. M. (1979). *Prediction of successful nursing performance* (Parts III and IV, Publication No. HRA 79–15). Washington, DC: Department of Health, Education, and Welfare.

Sealy, P. (1987). *Canadian masters' students in nursing experiences with the mentor relationship.* Unpublished master's thesis, University of Western Ontario, London. Canada.

Shields, D. A. (1986). *Mentoring relationships.* Unpublished master's thesis, Wright State University, Dayton, Ohio.

Slagle, J. C. (1986). The process of mentoring in nursing: A study of protégés' perceptions of the mentor–protégé relationship. (Doctoral dissertation, Teachers College, Columbia University). *Dissertation Abstracts International, 47,* 2377B.

Smith, L. A. (1985). Mentoring outcomes following nursing orientation programs in a critical care/teaching hospital. (Doctoral dissertation, George Peabody College, Vanderbilt University). *Dissertation Abstracts International, 46,* 3258A.

Smith, P. C., Kimball, L. K., & Hulin, C. L. (1969). *The measurement of satisfaction in work and retirement.* Chicago: Rand McNally.

Spengler, C. D. (1982). Mentor-protégé relationships: A study of career development among female nurse doctorates. (Doctoral dissertation, University of Missouri, Columbia). *Dissertation Abstracts International, 44,* 2113B.

Stogdill, R. M. (1963). *Manual for the Leader Behavior Description Questionnaire— Form XII: An experimental revision.* Columbus, OH: The Ohio State University, Bureau of Business Research.

Super, D. E. (1957). *The psychology of careers.* New York: Harper & Row.

Super, D. E., Crites, J., Hummel, R., Moser, H., Overstreet, P. L., & Warnath, C. (1957). *Vocational development: A framework for research.* New York: Teachers College Press.

Tagg, M. I. (1986). Mentoring in nursing: A study of the career development of professional nurse faculty in selected colleges of nursing. (Doctoral dissertation, Memphis State University). *Dissertation Abstracts International, 47,* 4826B.

Taylor, A. J. (1984). *Mentoring among nurse administrators.* Unpublished postmaster's study, British Columbia Institute of Technology, Vancouver.

Taylor, A. J. (1986). Mentoring among nurse administrators. In W. A. Gray & M. M. Gray (Eds.). *Proceedings of the First International Conference on Mentoring, II* (pp. 169–176). Vancouver, BC: International Association for Mentoring.

Vance, C. N. (1977). A group profile of contemporary influentials in American nursing. (Doctoral dissertation, Teachers College, Columbia University). *Dissertation Abstracts International, 38,* 4734B.

Vance, C. N. (1982). The mentor connection. *The Journal of Nursing Administration, 12*(4), 7–13.

Vance, C. N. (1986). The role of mentorship in the leadership development of nurse-influentials. In W. A. Gray and M. M. Gray (Eds.). *Proceedings of the First International Conference on Mentoring, II* (pp. 117–184). Vancouver, BC: International Association for Mentoring.

Vogt, R. B. (1985). The relationship of mentoring activity and career success of nursing faculty. (Doctoral dissertation, Northern Illinois University, DeKalb.) *Dissertation Abstracts International, 47,* 439A.

Ward, M. J., & Fetter, M. E. (1979). *Instruments for use in nursing education and research.* Boulder, CO: Western Interstate Commission for Higher Education.

Weiss, D. J., Davis, R. V., England, G. W., & Lofquist, L. H. (1967). *Manual for the Minnesota Satisfaction Questionnaire.* Minneapolis: University of Minnesota.

Werley, H. H., & Newcomb, B. J. (1983). The research mentor: A missing element in nursing? In N. L. Chaska (Ed.) *The nursing profession: A time to speak* (pp. 202–215). New York: McGraw-Hill.

White, J. F. (1986). The perceived role of mentoring in the career development and success of academic nurse administrators. (Doctoral dissertation, University of Pittsburgh.) *Dissertation Abstracts International, 47,* 1947A.

White, J. F. (1988). The perceived role of mentoring in the career development and success of academic nurse-administrators. *Journal of Professional Nursing, 4,* 178–185.

Williams, R. S. (1986). Relationship of mentoring by senior faculty to the productivity of junior faculty in the top twenty colleges of nursing in the United States. (Doctoral dissertation, The University of Michigan, Ann Arbor). *Dissertation Abstracts International, 47,* 3682A.

Williams, R. S., & Blackburn, R. T. (1988). Mentoring and junior faculty productivity. *Journal of Nursing Education, 27,* 204–209.

Wood, C. A. (1990). Baccalaureate nursing faculty perceptions of the mentoring activity of immediate supervisors. (Doctoral dissertation, The University of Mississippi, Tupelo). *Dissertation Abstracts International, 51,* 1927A.

Young, C. F. (1985). Women as protégé's: The perceptual development of female doctoral students who have completed their initial mentor–protégé relationship. (Doctoral dissertation, Syracuse University.) *Dissertation Abstracts International, 47,* 1903A.

Zimmerman, L. M. (1983). Factors influencing career success of women in nursing. (Doctoral dissertation, University of Nebraska, Lincoln.) *Dissertation Abstracts International, 44,* 1065–1066B.

PART V

Other Research

Chapter 10

Nutritional Studies in Nursing

Noni L. Bodkin and Barbara C. Hansen
School of Nursing and
Department of Physiology
School of Medicine
University of Maryland

CONTENTS

Enteral Nutrition Research
Parenteral Nutrition Research
Nausea and Vomiting
Eating Disorders: Weight Loss and Weight Gain
Appetite and the Regulation of Food Intake
Miscellaneous Studies
Summary and Future Directions

There is growing acknowledgment of the importance of nutritional status to the overall health and well-being of the individual. Not only do nutritional factors impact single organs (brain, heart, muscle), body systems (gastrointestinal, cardiovascular, renal, skin, and others) are affected as well. Both physiological and behavioral aspects of nutrition are critical to nursing care. Since the late 1960s when the pioneering studies with total parenteral nutrition were carried out (Dudrick, Wilmore, Vars, & Rhoads, 1968), there has been an increasing awareness on the part of nurse clinicians and researchers as to the importance of adequate nutrition and the ability of the individual to obtain and assimilate the nutrients necessary to fulfill metabolic requirements. Further, there is a complex relationship between the environment and an individual's nutritional status; this relationship has been described as both cause and effect (Bayer, Bauers, & Kapp, 1983). An understanding of social and cultural factors related to appetite and hunger is essential in providing comprehensive patient care. Also essential is knowledge of the specific effects that illness and related therapies often have on the individual's emotional and physical well-being and thus nutritional status.

Multiple aspects of the concept and application of nutrition serve as potential key factors in the patient's illness, treatment, recovery, and subsequent health. Moore, Guenter, and Bender (1986) compiled an excellent review of the contributions of nurses to the nutrition research literature between 1970 and 1984. This chapter is focused on studies on nutritional issues carried out by nurses. The criteria for selection were studies that: (a) were carried out using the research process, (b) were concerned with nutrition or gastrointestinal related issues, and (c) had a nurse as the primary author. The studies were identified using both author- and subject-based computer searches of the literature from 1970 to 1989. The primary journals with the number of studies found noted in parentheses included *Journal of Parenteral and Enteral Nutrition* (11), *Nursing Research* (11), *Oncology Nursing Forum* (8), *Cancer Nursing* (6), *Communicating Nursing Research* (3), *Journal of Advanced Nursing* (3), *and Journal of Neuroscience Nursing* (3). Other journals with at least 2 published reports meeting the above criteria included *Heart and Lung, Journal of Comparative and Physiological Psychology, Nursing Times,* and *Physiology and Behavior.*

An overview of nursing research carried out in nutrition and nutrition-related areas within the context of the research process and according to selected evaluation criteria will be presented. A brief description of each study is followed by comments and analysis. Discussion of results and concepts presented by various investigators is integrated according to the similarity of subject matter and research question. Finally, future research directions are suggested.

ENTERAL NUTRITION RESEARCH

In recent years nutritional support has emerged as a specialty area in nursing with new opportunities for the professional nurse in practice, education, and research. Grant and Kennedy-Caldwell (1988) have compiled a thorough and timely volume reviewing the literature on nutritional support in nursing. For the purpose of reviewing research by nurses in the area of nutritional support, enteral nutrition has been defined as the provision of necessary nutrients or supplements by tube feeding when the patient with a normally functioning gastrointestinal tract is unable or unwilling to eat. In contrast, parenteral nutrition is the administration of nutrients by the central or peripheral intravenous route in patients with nonfunctioning gastrointestinal tracts or with gastrointestinal disorders (Griggs, 1988).

Studies having to do with enteral nutrition represented the largest group of nutrition-related research reports in nursing. Given that the administration of enteral feedings and assessment of patient response pose a significant challenge to the nurse in the clinical setting, this area is well-justified as a research focus.

B. C. Walike and J. W. Walike (1973; 1977) studied the lactose content of tube-feeding diets as a cause of diarrhea in patients principally diagnosed as having head and neck cancer. Using two identical liquid diets that differed only in the presence or absence of 7% lactose, 11 patients were studied in a double-blind cross-over experimental design for approximately 10 consecutive days per period. Outcome variables included stool frequency and consistency and the results of a lactose tolerance test.

The investigators (Walike & Walike, 1973, 1977) found that both stool frequency and consistency were significantly different on the two diets and concluded that the lactose content of liquid diets commonly used in tube feedings was a major cause of diarrhea. The choice of double-blind experimental study design, use of a clinical research unit with close monitoring of patients, and accurate intake/output records were noteworthy. The 1977 expansion of the study to include 16 subjects led to a firm recommendation by the authors to reduce or eliminate lactose from liquid diets.

Many of the studies related to nasogastric tube feeding (or enteral feeding, as it is now termed) were performed by the Tube Feeding Consortium. This group of researchers was among the first to combine their expertise to design and conduct a series of multicenter investigations in clinical nursing and chose to focus their attention on nursing problems associated with enteral feeding. The groundwork and justification for research in this area was laid by the initial group in its pilot study (Walike et al., 1974). In this preliminary study, issues and problems associated with nasogastric tube feeding were identified in an extensive survey of 121 enterally fed patients. Findings of the study included documentation of the frequency of common gastrointestinal responses to tube feeding including diarrhea, nausea, and vomiting. In addition, the effects of rate and temperature of feeding on body weight, and fluid and electrolyte balance were noted, as well as patient responses, attitudes and adjustments to enteral feeding. The data, collected retrospectively, were recorded on 145 variables for periods up to 20 days of tube feeding. This study provided convincing evidence that the nurse is in a unique position to assess and record patient responses to tube feedings and to modify the procedures to the patient's benefit. Further, the investigators documented several potential clinical problems with enteral nutrition that would be appropriate for future study. The findings were discussed further in two other reports (Hanson et al., 1975; Kubo et al., 1976).

Other studies, resulting directly from the initial consortium study,

included that of Williams and B. C. Walike (1975) who found that temperature of the tube feeding administered to a sample of rhesus monkeys had only
a brief and insignificant effect on gastric motility, with those minimal effects
limited to the first few minutes following the infusion. The authors concluded
that there were no deleterious effects of infusing liquid diets in a temperature
range of 5° to 37°C. The use of rhesus monkeys, whose gastrointestinal tract
resembles that of humans, and gastric recording devices which allowed
physiological measurements, lent significance to the findings. These findings
were consistent with those of Hanson (1973) who studied 5 normal, healthy
adult volunteers, and demonstrated that warming a tube feeding (when 250
mL is given over ≥30 minutes) is a nursing procedure that lacks scientific
support; he found no difference between the temperatures of the warmed and
cold feedings on reaching the stomach. The temperature of the tube feeding in
the stomach was measured using a Thermester probe placed in the lumen of
the nasogastric tube. The sensor tip of the probe was located at the distal end
of the tube.

In a later study, the group, now enlarged in number of investigators
(Kagawa-Busby, Heitkemper, Hansen, Hanson, & Vanderburg, 1980), again
addressed the effect of different temperatures of tube feeding on gastric
motility, transit time, and patient response in 6 healthy adults. Intragastric
measurements of gastric motility and temperature (via the feeding tube) and
stool markers were utilized. The investigators found that a refrigerated formula (allowed to come to room temperature) or a commercially packaged
(nonrefrigerated) formula could be administered without distress to the
patient.

Regarding patient responses to tube feedings, Padilla et al. (1979)
attempted to identify the subjective distresses of nasogastric feeding in 30
hospitalized patients. A 47-item interview schedule was used. Among several
psychosensory disturbances, the most common distressing experiences
associated with tube feeding included "feeling thirsty" and "being deprived of
good tasting food." This report included a good discussion of specific nurs-
ing-related interventions to alleviate or prevent the psychosensory disturbances identified.

In another physiologically oriented study, Heitkemper, Martin, Hansen,
Hanson, and Vanderburg (1981) measured the effects of feeding volume and
rate of delivery on gastric pressure and subject tolerance. The authors found
that in initiating feedings the first feeding was best given slowly (30 mL/min)
and in a small volume (350 mL or less); adverse symptoms decreased and
tolerance improved with repeated feedings. In a later study, Heitkemper and
Hansen (1984) showed that gastric relaxation associated with infusion of a
liquid meal could be conditioned to auditory cues, lead to decreased intragastric pressure, and thus have significant effects on gastric function.

The risk of pulmonary aspiration in patients receiving tube feedings is a concern, particularly in patients with a depressed level of consciousness, artificial airways, or continuous feedings. At least two groups (Elpern, Jacobs, & Bone, 1987; Treloar & Stechniller, 1984) have evaluated the incidence of pulmonary aspiration; conflicting results were obtained. Both research teams used methylene blue dye as an indication of aspiration. A similar number of subjects ($N = 31$ in Elpern et al. and 30 in Treloar & Stechniller) were followed; however, Elpern et al. monitored subjects every 4 hours by assessment of tracheal secretions obtained from suctioning. In contrast, Treloar and Stechniller assessed the color and character of the tracheal aspirate every 12 hours. This difference in study design may have influenced the findings, as Elpern et al. found a 27% incidence of aspiration (247 of 907 aspirate samples) while the latter group found no evidence of aspiration. Additional studies are warranted.

Taylor (1982) and Kocan and Hickisch (1986) addressed the incidence of diarrhea and aspiration in patients receiving continuous versus intermittent tube feedings. Several related factors were considered, including medications, size and type of nasogastric tube, size and type of tracheostomy or endotracheal tube, and level of consciousness. In the two studies aspiration and diarrhea occurred with both methods of tube feeding administration; there were no significant differences in regard to level of consciousness, frequency or consistency of stools, incidence of antibiotic use, incidence of aspiration, amount of residual gastric contents, and amount of nursing time required by the subjects. The Kocan and Hickisch report included a thoughtful discussion that addressed each of the study objectives and findings. The investigators noted that no one method was best suited for all patients; rather, nutritional therapy must be tailored to meet the needs of the individual.

Metheny, Spies, and Eisenberg (1986) studied the frequency of nasoenteral tube displacement and associated risk factors in 105 subjects over a 6-month period. The investigators found that 92% of the tubes ($N = 213$) in use were of the small-bore variety in contrast to the once popular firm, large-bore tubes. The most frequent complication was spontaneous dislocation. Intubation and suctioning of the upper airway were risk factors that were significant in the displacement of unweighted intestinal tubes, as were a decreased level of consciousness, retching, and vomiting. Failure to elevate the head of the bed did not predispose to tube displacement, nor did the use of round-the-clock narcotics. The large sample and objective data recording, including the use of radiographic reports, lent confidence to the results of this study.

A number of investigators have addressed technical issues involved in nasogastric feeding. As the administration of tube feedings is clearly a nursing responsibility, this is a potential area for determining the scientific basis for various steps and precautions commonly taken in the feeding procedure.

One of the studies most applicable to the clinical setting was that of

Hanson (1979) who identified noninvasive criteria for predicting the proper length of the nasogastric tube prior to insertion. Other recent studies of technical interest include the evaluation of a new polyurethane feeding tube (Crocker, Krey, & Steffee, 1981), in which subjects were used as their own controls and an evaluation of four holding devices for securing feeding tubes (McDonald, Williams, Daggett, Schut, Swint, & Buckwalter, 1982).

Schroeder, Fisher, Volz, and Paloucek (1983) and Gibbs (1983) both carried out well-designed studies of microbial contamination of tube feedings and the origin of such contamination. The researchers of both studies identified significant numbers and types of bacterial contamination. These studies were innovative and objective, as the authors sought to identify pathogenic sources by bacterial culture of equipment and formulas in both the clinical setting and the diet kitchen.

PARENTERAL NUTRITION RESEARCH

Only a small percentage of all nutrition studies conducted by nurses were in the area of parenteral nutrition. However, those identified were of particular value in regard to study design and data collection.

DeSomery and Walike (1976) and Hansen, DeSomery, Hagedorn, and Kalnasy (1977) studied the effect of parenteral nutrition on gastric motility, voluntary food intake, and appetite suppression in monkeys. The purpose of these studies was to investigate the effects of parenteral nutrition on appetite during and following the conclusion of parenteral nutrition.

The authors of both studies found that administration of parenteral nutrition in caloric amounts equal to normal intake resulted in a significant decrease in oral intake, possibly accounting for the lack of appetite observed in many patients. In addition, when oral intake and weight gain are desirable during parenteral nutrition, infusing the diet in amounts less than baseline may result in a higher total caloric intake than parenteral nutrition alone as the patient may have less suppression of appetite. Finally, oral intake continued to be decreased even when parenteral nutrition was discontinued for a period of time.

Although the sample size ($N = 2$) was a limitation of the earlier study, 9 monkeys were used in the latter study and lend credence to the findings. The use of nonhuman primates in both studies allowed the control of multiple influences on appetite (e.g., learning, emotions, and social patterns) that often are significant confounding factors in humans. In addition, the liquid diet permitted accurate measurement of oral intake and the physiological measurements of gastric motility concurrent with parenteral and oral intake warrants added confidence in the findings.

More recently, Martyn, Hansen, and Jen (1984) also studied the effects of parenteral nutrition on food intake and gastric motility in monkeys. Periods of parenteral nutrition of different levels (25, 50, 75, and 100% of baseline caloric intake) were alternated with periods without parenteral nutrition (oral food intake was provided ad libitum). The investigators replicated and extended earlier research in this area. The findings were similar to those previously described.

Addressing more technical details of parenteral nutrition, Jarrard, Olson, and Freeman (1980) carried out a prospective study of the effects of daily subclavian dressing changes on the incidence of catheter-related sepsis in hospitalized patients. They found that when dressings were changed daily, no positive skin or blood cultures were found during 242 patient days, in contrast to a 3.5% incidence of positive skin cultures over 530 patient days in the group undergoing Monday-Wednesday-Friday dressing changes.

Guenter, Moore, Crosby, Buzby, and Mullen (1982) conducted a retrospective review of patient medical records to determine compliance with requirements for daily weight measurements in patients receiving parenteral and enteral nutrition. They found that daily weights were recorded in only 65.5% of the patients undergoing parenteral therapy and 53% of patients undergoing enteral therapy. In addition, a semi-structured questionnaire was administered to the nursing staff to attempt to determine nursing perceptions of reasons for not obtaining body weight measurements as ordered. Only 68% of the nursing staff considered weights very important. Reasons given for failure to weigh were: (a) patient too ill, (2) other priorities, and (3) patient refused to be weighed.

NAUSEA AND VOMITING

The incidence of nausea and vomiting has been the focus of several nursing studies in a number of different clinical areas. DiIorio (1985) was concerned with the effectiveness of nonpharmacological treatments to control nausea and vomiting in pregnant teenagers and attempted to determine those treatments most effective. The sample consisted of 92 subjects (primarily 17 to 19 year olds) attending three county health department maternity clinics; of these, 78 completed questionnaires. Fifty-six percent of the subjects experienced nausea and vomiting; these findings were similar to previous reports of a 55% to 72% incidence (Brandes, 1967; Wolkind & Zajicek, 1978). In addition, DiIorio found that white teenagers were more likely than black teenagers to experience nausea/vomiting and that girls who wanted the pregnancy were more likely to have experienced nausea/vomiting than those who did not. This study was strengthened by the use of a 6th-grade reading level questionnaire and the establishment of content validity.

Several studies have been carried out to identify the incidence of nausea and vomiting in cancer patients, associated factors, and effective treatments. Welch (1980) studied nausea and vomiting in patients undergoing external beam radiotherapy and Seipp, Chang, Shiling, and Rosenberg (1980) compared delta-9-tetrahydrocannabinol (THC) to placebo for the control of nausea and vomiting in patients receiving high-dose methotrexate.

In the latter study, the authors noted that during the course of the study, it appeared that the double-blind design was not being maintained, and the participants (both nurses and patients) were able to identify which drug was being administered. A survey was then given to the nurses on the unit to obtain information regarding their attitudes toward participation in the project and the use of marijuana. The authors found that 95% (19 of 20) respondents believed the study was appropriate because conventional antiemetics had been unsuccessful in this patient group. Most of the staff (70%) felt they were adequately prepared for the project but viewed the study with apprehension. A follow-up survey conducted 1 year later showed that attitudes of the staff were essentially unchanged. However, due to a staffing shortage, the nurses found the hourly rating scales more difficult to complete. The authors concluded that unfavorable bias on the part of the nursing staff was unlikely. For future study, the authors recommended substituting a phenothiazine-like compound or tranquilizer rather than the inert placebo.

Kennedy, Packard, Grant, and Padilla (1981) noted that both oncology nurses and patients have found nausea and vomiting to be one of the most distressing side effects of chemotherapy. These investigators used a questionnaire approach to survey both nurses and patients from 18 hospitals and medical centers across the United States as to occurrence of nausea/vomiting, causes, and treatment approaches. Nausea and vomiting were the most common side effects of chemotherapy. From 64 nurse (39% response rate) and 115 patient (25% response rate) questionnaires, the investigators determined that antiemetics, various foods and drinks (crackers, ginger ale, etc.), and various forms of distraction (music, relaxation techniques, etc.) were the interventions most often reported as helpful by both nurses and patients.

Daniels and Belt (1982) and Gathercole, Connolly, and Birdsell (1982) studied the use of metoclopramide and dexamethasone, respectively, as antiemetic adjuncts in patients receiving chemotherapy. In the study by Daniels and Belt, 31 adult patients received 55 treatments of metoclopramide and cisplatinum. The authors reported a complete absence of nausea and vomiting in 30 courses (55%) of treatment (21 patients). Interestingly, 9 of the patients who had also received 13 courses of chemotherapy without metoclopramide treatment had a 100% incidence of nausea and vomiting. In addition, side effects of metoclopramide were few in number and not severe (drowsiness and mild, short-term diarrhea). The authors included specific recommendations and helpful guidelines for metoclopramide administration.

In the study by Gathercole (1982) and associates, 20 patients undergoing chemotherapy were given dexamethasone as an antiemetic agent. The investigators found that dexamethasone significantly decreased the incidence of nausea and vomiting. The investigators noted that the double-blind aspect of the study was lost when the side effects of the dexamethasone (rectal tingling or generalized tingling) became known to the patients.

Moore (1982) investigated the influence of the time of administration of chemotherapy on nausea and vomiting in 13 adult patients. In this study, no significant relationship was found between time of chemotherapy administration and nausea and vomiting; therefore, the data did not support the nursing observation that chemotherapy administered during the evening hours would be less likely to result in nausea and vomiting because the patients "sleep off" their symptoms. The author noted that the small sample size, nonrandom sampling, and lack of experimental control over antiemetic therapy (type or administration) were limitations of the study.

Cotanch (1983) and Frank (1985) used relaxation and distraction techniques as treatment approaches to decrease the anxiety associated with the nausea and vomiting in patients undergoing chemotherapy. In the study by Cotanch, 9 of 12 patients showed a decrease in nausea and vomiting following muscle relaxation training. Similarly, Frank provided evidence that in 15 patients using music therapy and guided visual imagery, the perception and occurrence of nausea was not significantly decreased, although the degree of vomiting and length of vomiting were significantly decreased. Both Cotanch and Frank indicated that creative strategies for decreasing chemotherapy-induced nausea and vomiting warranted further study.

Rhodes, Watson, and Johnson (1984; 1985) carried out a series of studies of nausea and vomiting in chemotherapy patients. These investigations were designed to develop an instrument that would measure the patient's perception of nausea and vomiting; in a later study (1986) they described the relationship of anxiety to nausea and vomiting during consecutive cycles of chemotherapy. The studies were somewhat limited by small sample sizes (32, 32, and 36), the lack of control of antiemetics and other medications, differing cycles of chemotherapy, and patient dropout. Recommendations for further research with a larger sample size under a longitudinal design were included.

Dixon (1984) attempted to integrate several noninvasive nursing interventions as a treatment approach to the cachexia of cancer. Of the initial 88 patients, only 55 were able to remain in the study for the entire 4-month intervention program. The author concluded that progressive nutritional deterioration often associated with cancer could be slowed effectively by home-based nursing intervention. Suggestions for further research were noted.

EATING DISORDERS: WEIGHT LOSS AND WEIGHT GAIN

In the area of eating disorders and weight loss, a number of studies have been carried out, both physiological and behavioral in nature. Wang and Watson (1978) were among the first to address the question of successful weight reduction in obesity; they described contingency contracting with an obese adolescent. Wineman (1980), Mallick (1982), and Gierszewski (1983) used questionnaires to study obesity, weight loss, body image, and locus of control in obese subjects undertaking weight loss classes or programs. In particular, Mallick sought to identify health problems associated with dieting in adolescent females and found that hunger, weakness, headaches, and fatigue were reported most frequently.

In a unique approach, White (1984) addressed the relationship of nursing practice and research by identifying a clinical problem, carrying out the research, and then using the research findings in practice. The clinical problem was to identify high-risk clients and decrease client attrition in an obesity program. Using the findings of the investigation, the attrition rate in the program decreased from 50% to 10%. This investigator illustrated how a nurse can use the research process to study a clinical problem and, very importantly, apply the findings to the clinical setting with a positive outcome on nursing practice.

A number of investigators (Laffrey, 1986; Orr, 1985; Price, O'Connell, and Kulkulka, 1985) have used questionnaires and knowledge scales to investigate knowledge of obesity and its consequences, caloric content of food, weight loss techniques, and perceived health status in adult volunteers and college students, both normal and overweight. In general, many of the respondents were poorly informed as to the above-noted areas. Laffrey emphasized the importance of understanding and incorporating the clients' perceived health status into the treatment approach in order to meet their health needs successfully. Similarly, Jones, Doheny, Jones, and Bradley (1986) addressed the problem of binge-eating in college students. Using a questionnaire, the researchers showed a high prevalence of bulimia in the young, female, middle-income population. Many subjects, however, described frequent binge episodes but did not consider themselves to have an eating disorder.

At least two studies of weight gain during various therapeutic situations have been reported. Harris and Eth (1981) studied 123 patients admitted to an adult inpatient psychiatric ward to receive acute treatment (average length of stay 27 days). Seventy two (59%) of the 123 patients were treated with one or more neuroleptic medications during their hospitalization. A control group of 30 unmedicated patients was included. Of the patients on neuroleptic medication, 63% showed weight gain of 2.0 to 2.3 kg and 37% showed no weight gain. Of the control group, 53% had a mean weight gain of 0.4 kg. The authors concluded that patients receiving neuroleptic medication tend to gain weight and the increased body weight might be related to the length of treatment. Following the study, patient education on the unit was altered to note the possibility of weight gain as a side effect of the treatment and to include suggestions as to weight gain prevention.

Foltz (1985) studied weight gain among stage II breast cancer patients prior to initiation and at completion of chemotherapy in 34 women. Several data collection tools, both physiological and behavioral, were used, including psychiatric scales for activity and depression, indirect calorimetry for resting metabolic rate, radioimmunoassay for serum estradiol, 24-hr recall for food intake, and measurements of body weight. The author found that changes in depression activity, resting metabolic rate, and oral intake were not significantly different between patients who gained weight and those who did not. Serum estradiol was reduced significantly among weight-gaining women in comparison to women not gaining weight; however, no relationship was identified between the reduced estradiol level and either increased intake or decreased activity. Further research was suggested.

In regard to additional studies in oncology patients, the problem of weight loss has been addressed by Johnston, Keane, and Prudo (1982) and Mayer, Hetrick, Riggs, and Sherwin (1984). Both sets of investigators used nutritional and physiological indices and documented significant weight loss in patients undergoing radiation therapy for head and neck cancer and patients receiving recombinant leukocyte A interferon. In addition, documentation of the pattern of weight loss as related to the stages of therapy and the onset and severity of gastrointestinal side effects provided a basis for nursing-initiated nutritional interventions and support.

APPETITE AND THE REGULATION OF FOOD INTAKE

Several nurse researchers have addressed appetite and the regulation of food intake in humans through physiological research. In the earliest of these included here because it was one of the original research studies in nursing, Walike, Jordan, and Stellar (1969a; 1969b) proposed to study some of the behavioral and physiological factors controlling caloric ingestion in humans.

In a laboratory setting, 21 subjects were studied for breakfast or lunch 3 to 5 times a week for periods ranging from 6 to 45 weeks. The subjects ingested a well-balanced liquid diet (Metrecal, 0.97 cal/mL) over 20 minutes. The effect of various sizes of preloads on subsequent ingestion, ratings of hunger, and estimates of intake were determined. The preload was a volume of liquid diet taken from a glass by the subject, usually within one minute and prior to subject volume ingestion. The investigator found that subjects consistently decreased the amount of diet taken through the straw as the size of preload increased; however, the subjects did not decrease the amounts sufficiently to prevent overeating. A trial of voluntary intragastric feeding (whereby the diet was either pumped into the mouth or delivered via a nasogastric tube) showed that subjects ingested stable daily intakes (approximating their baseline oral intake) after an initial period of adaptation. The provision of oral, in addition to gastric, intake appeared to increase the tendency of the subjects to overeat. In contrast, when the meal was delivered entirely intragastrically to a subset of 4 of the subjects, one subject greatly reduced his intake below baseline, while the other 3 subjects ingested amounts approximating their oral intake.

The investigators proposed using the method of preloads, oral and/or voluntary intragastric feeding for the objective study of feeding behavior in humans. They concluded that these studies demonstrated the consistency of short-term regulation of appetite during experimental meals that can be deregulated by certain manipulations (rapid ingestion, lack of oral cues, simultaneous oral and intragastric feeding).

Additional studies by Hansen et al. (Hansen, Jen, & Brown, 1981; Hansen, Jen, & Kalnasy, 1981; Walike [Hansen] & Smith, 1972) have used the rhesus monkey *(Macaca mulatta)* for the study of the regulation of food intake, meal pattern, and body weight, allowing the detailed assessment of both behavioral and physiological parameters involved in the regulation of food intake. Metzger and Hansen (1983) also used the rhesus monkey ($N = 4$) to study the effect of cholecystokinin on feeding, glucose, and pancreatic hormones. They found that infusing an intravenous dose of cholecystokinin at the beginning of the meal significantly decreased food intake and delayed plasma glucose and insulin responses over 3 hours. The use of simultaneous free-feeding and intragastric infusions in these studies permitted the assessment of nutrient alteration of the diet without the confounding effects of palatability.

In a unique study, Heitkemper and Marotta (1985) proposed that specific diet manipulation (composition or quantity) would produce central nervous system alterations. Using a rat model ($N = 15$), these researchers showed that dietary manipulation of one neurotransmitter (choline) produced significant decreases in adrenergic but not cholinergic enzyme activity in the gastrointestinal tract. Particularly in prolonged fasting, alertness to disturbances in gastrointestinal function and early intervention are indicated.

MISCELLANEOUS STUDIES

In the area of nutritional assessment, only 2 nursing studies were identified. Layton, Gallucci, & Aker (1981) conducted a comprehensive investigation to address the nutritional status of 8 allogeneic bone marrow recipients receiving total parenteral nutrition. Several nutritional parameters were measured at regular intervals. The investigators found that total parenteral nutrition administered to all patients had an overall positive effect but was insufficient to prevent the decreased nutritional status of the subjects. The authors speculated that, without total parenteral nutrition, even more severe malnutrition would have occurred, but in the way administered, total parenteral nutrition did not prevent nutritional decline in patients.

Jones, Moore, and Van Way (1983) sought to reconcile the discrepancy between the prognostic nutritional index (predictive of the risk of morbidity and mortality in elective surgery) with the abdominal trauma index (used for intraoperative scoring of abdominal injuries) in regard to predicting postoperative morbidity and mortality in acute trauma patients. In 24 patients undergoing emergency laparotomy for acute abdominal trauma, the investigators found that the prognostic nutritional index was altered by blood loss and therefore was less reliable in predicting complications following trauma.

Specific diet therapy as a treatment modality for various disorders has been addressed by a few nurse researchers. Davis (1978) investigated the dietary pathogenesis of schizophrenia under the hypothesis that a gluten-free diet would be of value in improving chronic schizophrenia. All patients were started with a gluten-free diet for an 18-week period using a double-blind cross-over experimental design. The author noted that the results were not conclusive. The number of patients studied was not clear. The author noted that, of the patients participating, the condition of one of the males and one of the females remained primarily unchanged.

Kinney and Blount (1979) studied the effect of ingestion of large amounts of cranberry juice on the urinary pH of healthy humans ($N = 40$) ingesting a controlled diet. In daily amounts ranging from 450 to 720 mL, cranberry juice (in an 80% concentration) was associated with significantly decreased urinary pH. The benefits of this decreased pH and bacteriostatic effects as well as the limitations of the study were discussed.

SUMMARY AND FUTURE DIRECTIONS

The substantial contribution that nurses have made in the area of nutritional research is apparent from this review. In regard to research questions, the majority of studies were focused on enteral nutrition and nausea/vomiting, with a lesser number of studies related to parenteral nutrition, eating disorders, appetite, and body weight gain or loss.

Although most of the studies reviewed were carried out by single researchers or groups of two or three researchers who addressed a single question, the Tube Feeding Consortium (which initially included Walike et al., 1974) set forth to design and conduct a series of multi-center investigations on enteral feeding. A number of timely and key studies and reports resulted from the initial consortium study.

Due to the close interaction of multiple physiological, psychological, environmental, and cultural factors in the regulation of appetite and feeding, and ultimately the nutritional status, the selection of instruments and methods for research in this area is of particular importance. Quantitative and objective tools to measure these factors singly or in combination must be reliable and valid. In addition, such tools must have a degree of simplicity and directness to facilitate a realistic and feasible study design. As outlined in this review, nurses have used a wide variety of instruments and methods in nutrition-related research. Replication of studies is warranted not only to validate previous results but also to establish appropriate methodologies.

Studies of particular relevance to clinical practice included those of Hanson (1979), who developed a method for proper placement of feeding tubes; Walike and Walike (1973; 1977) regarding lactose intolerance; White (1984), who developed an obesity program; Treloar and Stechmiller (1984) and Elpern et al. (1987), who studied the incidence of pulmonary aspiration and associated factors in patients receiving tube feedings; and Schroeder et al. (1983) and Gibbs (1983), who conducted studies to identify the source and extent of microbial contamination of tube feedings. Due to the significance of the findings and the potential benefits to the patient, it is recommended that these studies and their results be examined carefully with respect to utility and implementation in practice.

Some issues for further study include the psychological/emotional effects of enteral/parenteral nutrition, procedure-related issues in enteral/parenteral nutrition (incidence and prevention of complications, dressing changes, and optimal delivery of nutrients), effective interventions for prevention and control of nausea and vomiting, promotion of optimal body weight, and nutritional assessment tools. In addition, the growing number of persons with acquired immunodeficiency syndrome (AIDS) and the frequent, significant number of these clients who will have gastrointestinal involvement and dysfunction, present nurses with the challenge of identifying effective nutritional interventions and therapies. Finally, decision making, family and patient support, and ethical issues relating to hydration and nutrition in the care of terminally ill patients have not been addressed and remain a critical concern in nursing practice.

REFERENCES

Bayer, L. M., Bauers, C. M., & Kapp, S. R. (1983). Psychosocial aspects of nutritional support. *Nursing Clinics of North America, 18,* 119–128.

Brandes, J. M. (1967). First trimester nausea and vomiting as related to outcome of pregnancy. *Obstetrics and Gynecology, 30,* 427–431.

Cotanch, P. H. (1984). Relaxation training for control of nausea and vomiting in patients receiving chemotherapy. *Cancer Nursing, 6,* 277–283.

Crocker, K. S., Krey, S. H., & Steffee, W. P. (1981). Performance evaluation of a new nasogastric feeding tube. *Journal of Parenteral and Enteral Nutrition, 5,* 80–82.

Daniels, M. & Belt, R. J. (1982). High dose metoclopramide as an antiemetic for patients receiving chemotherapy with cis-platinum. *Oncology Nursing Forum, 9,* 20–22.

Davis, C. (1978, December 7). Dietary pathogenesis of schizophrenia. *Nursing Times, 74*(49), 2020–2021.

DeSomery, C. H., & Walike, B. C. (1976). Effects of parenteral nutrition on voluntary food intake and gastric motility in monkeys. In M. Batey (Ed.), *Communicating nursing research* (Vol. 8, pp. 176–187). Boulder, CO: Western Interstate Commission for Higher Education.

DiIorio, C. (1985). First trimester nausea in pregnant teenagers: Incidence, characteristics, intervention. *Nursing Research, 34,* 372–374.

Dixon, J. (1984). Effect of nursing interventions on nutritional and performance status in cancer patients. *Nursing Research, 33,* 330–335.

Dudrick, S. J., Wilmore, D. W., Vars, H. M., & Rhoads, J. E. (1968). Long-term total parenteral nutrition with growth, development, and positive nitrogen balance. *Surgery, 64,* 134–142.

Elpern, E. H., Jacobs, E. R., & Bone, R. C. (1987). Incidence of aspiration in tracheally intubated adults. *Heart & Lung, 16,* 527–531.

Foltz, A. T. (1985). Weight gain among stage II breast cancer patients: A study of five factors. *Oncology Nursing Forum, 12*(3), 21–26.

Frank, J. M. (1985). The effects of music therapy and guided visual imagery on chemotherapy induced nausea and vomiting. *Oncology Nursing Forum, 12,* 47–52.

Gathercole, F., Connolly, N., & Birdsell, J. (1982). The use of dexamethasone (hexadrol) as an antiemetic in association with chemotherapy for neoplastic disease. *Oncology Nursing Forum, 9,* 17–19.

Gibbs, J. (1983, February 16). Bacterial contamination of nasogastric feeds. *Nursing Times, 79*(7), 41–47.

Gierszewski, S. A. (1983). The relationship of weight loss, locus of control, and social support. *Nursing Research, 32,* 43–47.

Grant, J. A., & Kennedy-Caldwell, C. (1988). *Nutritional support in nursing.* Philadelphia: Grune and Statton.

Griggs, B. A. (1988). Indications for nutritional support in the adult patient. In Grant, J. A., & Kennedy-Caldwell, C. (Eds.), *Nutritional support in nursing* (pp. 65–89) Philadelphia: Grune and Statton.

Guenter, P. A., Moore, K., Crosby, L. O., Buzby, G. P., & Mullen, J. L. (1982). Body weight measurement of patients receiving nutritional support. *Journal of Parenteral and Enteral Nutrition, 6,* 441–443.

Hansen, B., DeSomery, C. H., Hagedorn, P. K., & Kalnasy, L. W. (1977). Effects of enteral and parenteral nutrition on appetite in monkeys. *Journal of Parenteral and Enteral Nutrition, 1,* 83–88.

Hansen, B. C., Jen, K-L. C., & Brown, N. (1981). Regulation of food intake and body weight in rhesus monkeys. In L. A. Cioffi, W. P. T. James, & T. B. Van Itallie (Eds.), *The body weight regulatory system: Normal and disturbed mechanisms.* New York: Raven Press.

Hansen, B. C., Jen, K-L. C., & Kalnasy, L. W. (1981). Control of food intake and meal patterns in monkeys. *Physiology and Behavior, 27,* 803–810.

Hanson, R. L. (1973). Effects of administering cold and warmed tube feedings. In M. V. Batey (Ed.), *Communicating nursing research* (Vol. 6, pp. 136–140). Boulder, CO: Western Interstate Commission for Higher Education.

Hanson, R. L. (1979). Predictive criteria for length of nasogastric tube insertion for tube feeding. *Journal of Parenteral and Enteral Nutrition, 3,* 160–163.

Hanson, R. L., Walike, B. C., Grant, M., Kubo, W., Bergstrom, N., Padilla, G., & Wong, H. L. (1975). Patient responses and problems associated with tube feeding. *Washington State Journal of Nursing, 47*(1), 9–13.

Harris, E., & Eth, S. (1981). Weight gain during neuroleptic treatment. *International Journal of Nursing Studies 18,* 171–175.

Heitkemper, M., & Hansen, B. C. (1984). Gastric relaxation prior to enteral feeding. *Journal of Parenteral and Enteral Nutrition, 8,* 682–684.

Heitkemper, M., & Marotta, S. F. (1985). Role of diets in modifying gastrointestinal neurotransmitter enzyme activity. *Nursing Research, 34,* 19–23.

Heitkemper, M. E., Martin, D. L., Hansen, B. C., Hanson, R., & Vanderburg, V. (1981). Rate and volume of intermittent enteral feeding. *Journal of Parenteral and Enteral Nutrition, 5,* 125–129.

Jarrard, M. M., Olson, C. M., & Freeman, J. B. (1980). Daily dressing change effects on skin flora beneath subclavian catheter dressings during total parenteral nutrition. *Journal of Parenteral and Enteral Nutrition, 4,* 391–392.

Johnston, C., Keane, T. J., & Prudo, S. M. (1982). Weight loss in patients receiving radical radiation therapy for head and neck cancer: A prospective study. *Journal of Parenteral and Enteral Nutrition, 6,* 399–402.

Jones, S. L., Doheny, M. O., Jones, P. K., & Bradley, N. (1986). Binge eaters: A comparison of eating patterns of those who admit to binging and those who do not. *Journal of Advanced Nursing, 11,* 545–552.

Jones, T. N., Moore, E. E., & Van Way, C. W. (1983). Factors influencing nutritional assessment in abdominal trauma patients. *Journal of Parenteral and Enteral Nutrition, 7,* 115–116.

Kagawa-Busby, K. S., Heitkemper, M. M., Hansen, B. C., Hanson, R. L., & Vanderburg, V. V. (1980). Effects of diet temperature on tolerance of enteral feedings. *Nursing Research, 29,* 276–280.

Kennedy, M., Packard, R., Grant, M. M., & Padilla, G. V. (1981). Chemotherapy related nausea and vomiting: A survey to identify problems and interventions. *Oncology Nursing Forum, 8,* 19–22.

Kinney, A. B., & Blount, M. (1979). Effect of cranberry juice on urinary pH. *Nursing Research, 28,* 287–290.

Kocan, M. J., & Hickisch, S. M. (1986). A comparison of continuous and intermittent enteral nutrition in NICU patients. *Journal of Neuroscience Nursing, 18,* 333–337.

Kubo, W., Grant, M., Walike, B., Bergstrom, N., Wong, H., Hanson, R., & Padilla, G. (1976). Fluid and electrolyte problems of tube-fed patients. *American Journal of Nursing, 76,* 912–916.

Laffrey, S. C. (1986). Normal and overweight adults: Perceived weight and health behavior characteristics. *Nursing Research, 35,* 173–177.

Layton, P. B., Gallucci, B. B., & Aker, S. N. (1981). Nutritional assessment of allogeneic bone marrow recipients. *Cancer Nursing, 4,* 127–135.

Mallick, M. J. (1982). Health problems associated with dieting activities of a group of adolescent females. *Western Journal of Nursing Research, 4,* 167–177.

Martyn, P. A., Hansen, B. C., & Jen, K-L. C. (1984). The effects of parenteral nutrition on food intake and gastric motility. *Nursing Research, 33,* 336–342.

Mayer, D., Hetrick, K., Riggs, C., & Sherwin, S. (1984). Weight loss in patients receiving recombinant leukocyte A interferon (IFL$_r$A): A brief report. *Cancer Nursing, 7,* 53–56.

McDonald, E., Williams, H., Daggett, M., Schut, B., Swint, E., & Buckwalter, K. C. (1982). A comparison of four holding devices for anchoring nasogastric tubes. *Journal of Neurosurgical Nursing, 14,* 90–93.

Metheny, N. A., Spies, M., & Eisenberg, P. (1986). Frequency of nasoenteral tube displacement and associated risk factors. *Research in Nursing & Health, 9,* 241–247.

Metzger, B. L., & Hansen, B. C. (1983). Cholecystokinin effects on feeding, glucose, and pancreatic hormones in rhesus monkeys. *Physiology and Behavior, 30,* 509–518.

Moore, J. M. (1982). The influence of the time of administration on cis-platinum induced nausea and vomiting. *Oncology Nursing Forum, 9,* 26–32.

Moore, M. C., Guenter, P. A., & Bender, J. H. (1986). Nutrition-related nursing research. *Image: Journal of Nursing Scholarship, 18,* 18–21.

Orr, J. (1985). Obesity. *Journal of Advanced Nursing, 10,* 71–78.

Padilla, G. V., Grant, M., Wong, H., Hansen, B. W., Hanson, R. L., Bergstrom, N., & Kubo, W. (1979). Subjective distresses of nasogastric tube feeding. *Journal of Parenteral and Enteral Nutrition, 3,* 53–57.

Price, J. H., O'Connell, J. K., & Kulkulka, G. (1985). Development of a short obesity knowledge scale using four different response formats. *Journal of School Health, 55,* 382–384.

Rhodes, V. A., Watson, P. M., & Johnson, M. H. (1984). Development of reliable and valid measures of nausea and vomiting. *Cancer Nursing, 7,* 33–41.

Rhodes, V. A., Watson, P. M., & Johnson, M. H. (1985). Patterns of nausea and vomiting in chemotherapy patients: a preliminary study. *Oncology Nursing Forum, 12,* 42–48.

Rhodes, V. A., Watson, P. M., & Johnson, M. H. (1986). Association of chemotherapy related nausea and vomiting with pretreatment and posttreatment anxiety. *Oncology Nursing Forum, 13,* 41–47.

Schroeder, P., Fisher, D., Volz, M., & Paloucek, J. (1983). Microbial contamination of enteral feeding solutions in a community hospital. *Journal of Parenteral and Enteral Nutrition 7,* 364–368.

Seipp, C. A., Chang, A. E., Shiling, D. J., & Rosenberg, S. A. (1980). In search of an effective antiemetic: A nursing staff participates in marijuana research. *Cancer Nursing, 3,* 271–276.

Taylor, T. T. (1982). A comparison of two methods of nasogastric tube feedings. *Journal of Neurosurgical Nursing, 14,* 49–55.

Treloar, D. M., & Stechmiller, J. (1984). Pulmonary aspiration in tube-fed patients with artificial airways. *Heart & Lung, 13,* 667–671.

Walike, B. C., Jordan, H. A., & Stellar, E. (1969a). Preloading and the regulation of food intake in man. *Journal of Comparative and Physiological Psychology, 68,* 327–333.

Walike, B. C., Jordan, H. A., & Stellar, E. (1969b). Studies of eating behavior. *Nursing Research, 18,* 108–113.

Walike, B. C., Padilla, G., Bergstrom, N., Hanson, R. L., Kubo, W., Grant, M., & Wong, H. L. (1974). Patient problems related to tube feeding. In M. V. Batey (Ed.), *Communicating nursing research* (Vol. 7, pp. 88–112). Boulder, CO: Western Interstate Commission for Higher Education.

Walike, B. C., & Smith, O. A. (1972). Regulation of food intake during intermittent and continuous cross circulation in monkeys *(Macaca mulatta). Journal of Comparative and Physiological Psychology, 80,* 372–381.

Walike, B. C., & Walike, J. W. (1973). Lactose content of tube feeding diets as a cause of diarrhea. *The Laryngoscope, 133,* 1109–1115.

Walike, B. C., & Walike, J. W. (1977). Relative lactose intolerance. A clinical study of tube-fed patients. *Journal of the American Medical Association, 238,* 948–951.

Wang, R. Y., & Watson, J. (1978). Contracting for weight reduction—making the sacrifices worthwhile. *American Journal of Maternal Child Nursing, 3,* 46–49.

Welch, D. A. (1980). Assessment of nausea and vomiting in cancer patients undergoing external beam radiotherapy. *Cancer Nursing, 3,* 365–371.

White, J. H. (1984). The relationship of clinical practice and research. *Journal of Advanced Nursing, 9,* 181–187.

Williams, K. R., & Walike, B. C. (1975). Effect of the temperature of tube feeding on gastric motility in monkeys. *Nursing Research, 24,* 4–9.

Wineman, N. M. (1980). Obesity: Locus of control, body image, weight loss and age-at-onset. *Nursing Research, 29,* 231–237.

Wolkind, S., & Zajicek, E. (1978). Psychosocial correlates of nausea and vomiting in pregnancy. *Journal of Psychosomatic Research, 22,* 1–5.

Chapter 11

Health Conceptualizations

Margaret A. Newman
School of Nursing
University of Minnesota

CONTENTS

The conceptualizations of health in nursing literature can be classified broadly within two major paradigms. The first is the *wellness–illness continuum,* a bipolar interactive portrayal of health and illness in myriad configurations ranging from high-level wellness to depletion of health (death). High-level wellness is further conceptualized as sense of wellbeing, life satisfaction, and quality of life. Movement toward the negative end of the continuum includes adaptation to disease and disability through various levels of functional ability. The wellness–illness conceptualization is supported by Keller's (1981) review of health literature and is consistent with the categories identified by Smith (1981) in her philosophical analysis of health. Research based on this paradigm conforms primarily to scientific methods that seek to control for contextual effects, provide the basis for causal explanations, and predict future outcomes.

The second paradigm characterizes health as a unidirectional *developmental phenomenon* of unitary patterning of person-environment. The developmental perspective of health has been present in the nursing literature since 1970 but was not identified clearly with health until the late 1970s and early 1980s. It has been conceptualized as expanding consciousness, pattern or meaning recognition, personal transformation, and, tentatively, self-actualization. With her assumption regarding the developing diversity of patterning of the human system across the life span, Rogers (1970) introduced the paradigm shift from viewing aging as "running out of steam" to viewing it as the "ability to purposefully transform the current context with all of its problems and contradictions . . ." (Reed, 1983, p. 19). This shift toward a developmental perspective has had clear implications for the way in which health is conceptualized. Although not endorsing the developmental perspective to the extent of Rogers and Reed, Pender (1987, p. 7) has stated that "Health is a manifestation of evolving patterns of person/environment interaction throughout the life span." Research within this paradigm seeks to address the dynamic whole of the health experience; however, methods to accomplish this objective are still in preliminary stages of development.

These two perspectives, the wellness–illness continuum and the developmental perspective, serve as the organizing framework for this review. With the exception of the background section on conceptualizations of health, the review is based on nursing research literature published in the United States between December 1982 and December 1988. It begins chronologically where Pender's 1984 review ended, but has a different conceptual focus. A computer search of nursing periodical literature as well as direct perusal of major nursing research journals was used to identify published reports, which were selected on the basis of the reviewer's judgment of their relevance to the above-described conceptualizations of health. For example, a study in which adaptation was identified as a major concept was included regardless of whether or not the investigator associated the study with any particular conceptualization of health.

The reviewer acknowledges the influence of her current health perspective, grounded in the developmental paradigm, on the interpretation and evaluation presented here. Ilya Prigogine's theory of dissipative structures (1976) has seemed particularly meaningful in interpretation of research findings; therefore reference to his work is made at several points in the review. According to this theory of dissipative structures, dynamic systems go through a process of normal, predictable fluctuation (a kind of maintenance function) until some chance event, either external or internal, forces a giant fluctuation that creates a chaotic situation. In this state of seeming disorganization it is impossible to predict the future of the system, but eventually the system assumes a new direction at a higher, more complex level of organization and resumes another period of rhythmic fluctuation.

Areas *not* reviewed include the following: health promotion/illness prevention, health policy, health economics, health delivery services, health knowledge, health beliefs, international health, women's health, child health, and family health. Also excluded are specific topics that have been addressed in separate reviews: social support, bereavement, stress, coping with surgery, and physiological parameters of health. Some research that included aspects of the above areas is reported because of its relevance to the topics of this review.

OVERVIEW OF NURSING CONCEPTUALIZATIONS OF HEALTH

Based on a philosophical investigation, Smith (1981) claimed that all the various conceptions of health could be accounted for in four types: (1) the eudaimonistic model, which includes general well-being and self-realization; (2) the adaptive model, which characterizes health as effective adaptation to the physical and social environment; (3) the role performance model, which equates health with the ability to perform effectively in relevant roles; and (4) the clinical model, which is based on health as the absence of disease or disability. These views, which have been conceptualized on a health continuum, represented the dominant paradigm for nursing theory and research, at least through the mid-1970s and into the 1980s. Roy's adaptation model and Johnson's behavioral model are exemplary of this perspective (Johnson, 1980; Roy, 1976).

Smith's conceptualization portrayed health on a positive–negative continuum from wellness to illness. She did not address the transformative notion of health stemming from the developmental perspective introduced in the nursing literature by Rogers (1970). An increasing number of nursing theorists and researchers have adopted a developmental view of health (Fitzpatrick, 1983; Newman, 1979, 1983, 1986; Parse, 1981; Reed, 1983; Stevenson, 1983; Woods, 1988).

Several theorists have explicated their views of the dominant paradigms of health in nursing, but consensus as to what they represent and how they are labeled is yet to be achieved. Newman (1986) has described the "old" paradigm as a health-illness continuum and the "new" paradigm as health as the evolving pattern of the whole. Parse (1987, p. 32) describes one view of health as being "a dynamic state and process of physical, psychological, social, and spiritual well-being," a kind of adding up of perspectives, which she called the totality paradigm. From this perspective, human beings are adapting organisms and may need assistance in striving toward optimal health, a view that corresponds to the wellness–illness conceptualization. Parse's own view, which she called the simultaneity paradigm, stemmed from

Rogerian assumptions (Rogers, 1970). Both Newman's evolving pattern of the whole and Parse's simultaneity paradigm are consistent with a developmental perspective of unitary patterning of person–environment.

Laffrey, Loveland-Cherry, and Winkler (1986) attempted to distinguish an absence of disease orientation from a health orientation. The former was referred to as the pathogenic paradigm and was characterized by a mechanistic view of human beings in good or bad working order, with health as freedom from disease. Their health paradigm depicted human beings as autonomous, responsible individuals with the potential for growth, with health as fluid and subjective and inclusive of disease as part of the life process. At first glance these designations seemed to represent separate paradigms, but closer scrutiny revealed them rather to be opposite ends of the wellness–illness polarization. The notion of well-being as a goal in their health paradigm, and the operationalization of health according to Smith's four models (Laffrey, 1986) rendered this conceptualization of health consistent with the continuum view.

Several theorists have extended Rogers' work by their own conceptualizations of health and pattern. Newman (1979; 1983; 1986) based her theory of health on the assumption of unitary patterning of person–environment, moving in the direction of greater complexity (Rogers, 1970), or toward higher, more inclusive levels of consciousness. Disease, if present, was considered a manifestation of the underlying patterning and, as such, reflective of the process of expanding consciousness. Movement, time, and space were identified as integral with consciousness in the developing pattern of person–environment. Consciousness was defined as the total informational capacity of the undivided living system, manifested in the ability of the system to interact with the environment. Based on the developmental perspective of Rogers (1970) and the theory of expanding consciousness of Newman (1979), Schorr (1983) incorporated death as a developmental phenomenon of life.

Parse (1981), also relying heavily on Rogers' assumptions of unitary patterning and increasing complexity, defined health as a personal process of living based on the individual's values and choices, which are reflected in patterns of increasing complexity. According to this conceptualization, health is a continuous process of transcendence. Fitzpatrick (1983), basing her life perspective model clearly on Rogers' theoretical assumptions, emphasized meaning within crisis situations as the major focus.

Categorization of other theorists' views on health is more ambiguous. Evans (1979) cited Rogers' views on the whole person, but her concept of health was based on a continuum from high-level wellness to total depletion of energy (death). She emphasized the importance of functional ability to adapt to a changing environment. Crawford (1982), also referring to Rogers, sought to advance the relevance of the concept of pattern in nursing, but shifted from a Rogerian perspective (Rogers, 1970) of evolving patterning to a Johnsonian perspective (Johnson, 1980) of patterns as the functional ability to achieve balance and stability in meeting bodily and interpersonal needs in the context of illness situations.

Campbell (1980, p. 15) proposed using self-awareness as a broad conceptual framework for a holistic approach to nursing. Self-awareness was defined as the "dynamic, conscious, continuous and active gaining of knowledge about the psychological, physical, environmental, and philosophical components of the inner self," as well as interactions between the self and the outer environment that create symbolic meaning and meaningful formulations, the basis for self-protection and self-enhancement. Campbell's model projected diminished self-awareness as impairment, increasing self-awareness as the process for preventing disease and impairment, and facilitating self-awareness as healing. This conceptualization approached the idea of health as expanding consciousness but maintained the positive–negative view of ability–disability.

Concerned with the prevailing emphasis on change in nursing theory, Hall (1981) argued instead for a view of health in which stability is the goal. She acknowledged that living systems are undergoing constant change but, citing the fact that one system often grows at the expense of another, emphasized the need for maintenance of the stability of the system. If Hall's points were considered in light of Prigogine's theory of dissipative structures (Prigogine, 1976), both stability and change could be seen as necessary stages of the rhythmic fluctuation to higher levels of organization.

Hollen (1981) sought to view health in a holistic way and considered health as the ability to control one's own environment. She proposed a model based on a continuum of functional ability and available choices and designated mobility and awareness as examples of health. Narayan and Joslin (1980), too, advocated a concept of health focused on the ability to interact with the environment. They emphasized growth and suggested the incorporation of crisis theory as support for this perspective. Depletion of health potential was seen as an inability to interact with internal and external forces.

Critical of extant nursing conceptualizations as portraying either a dichotomous, bipolar view of health or an incomplete synthesis that does not consider the clients' view, Tripp-Reimer (1984) offered a two-dimensional model stemming from an anthropological perspective. Health was seen as a state combining objective biomedical components with subjective, cultural components of beliefs and practices about illness. The model was helpful in determining the congruence–incongruence of the client's perception of health with the medical perspective but does not relinquish a dichotomous view; rather it increased the number and complexity of the categories.

Woods et al. (1988) addressed the meaning of health by surveying a large multiethnic sample of middle-aged women. The responses were classified in terms of Smith's four models (clinical, role performance, adaptive, eudaimonistic), resulting in a strong predominance of the eudaimonistic model. The findings were interpreted as fitting within Parse's totality paradigm, and, at the same time, consistent with Parse's position that health is each person's own experience of valuing and with Watson's (1985) unity of mind, body, and soul. Both Parse's and Watson's views are more consistent with the simultaneity paradigm.

Methodological issues regarding the study of health were addressed at a Wingspread Conference. Based on Pender's (1987) overview of conceptual issues in health and health promotion, Cox (1987) called for a "holistic paradigm" but included within that framework both empirical–analytic approaches for prediction and control and the need to study dynamic context- and time-dependent phenomena. Holistic was being used more to mean all-inclusive than to depict a particular paradigm. Conference participants reflected the view that a broad spectrum of methods was needed. Muhlenkamp (1987) noted the deficiencies of a reductionistic approach but at the same time called for the development of standardized levels of health. Norbeck (1987), although a proponent of an empirical–analytic approach, acknowledged the need for holistic methods and emphasized the need to distinguish which research questions demanded which method. Tripp-Reimer (1987) pointed out that a phenomenological approach is useful in the study of the experience and meaning of health but does not address prediction.

Other authors spoke to the merits of their particular approaches. Allen (1987) offered critical social theory as an alternative to the dominance–control perspective of empirical–analytic methods. He maintained that in experimental studies the expert's health values are substituted for the values of those being studied. The intent of critical social theory is to promote autonomy and responsibility in the participants, that is, the ability to participate and express themselves in an unconstrained way. Based on preliminary steps to describe the methodology of pattern identification, Newman (1987) asserted that pattern cannot be seen in quantity but rather in relationships, and that connectedness, context, and time are fundamental characteristics of pattern. Stevenson (1987), in summarizing conference discussions, stated that the study of health would benefit from a "holistic" approach. However, the meaning of this term remained ambiguous.

Reynolds (1988) conducted a review of 10 years of nursing research in which health was a variable with the purpose of determining how nurses characterize health. Based on the way health was operationalized and measured, she found that researchers most often characterized health as absence of illness, disability, or symptoms. Reynolds concluded that despite extensive urging within the discipline to conceptualize health in ways other than absence of disease, nursing research on health remains largely within the clinical and stability models, emphasizing "normal" physical and mental health states from which deviations may occur. The outcome of this review is similar. Although different paradigms are explicated, the predominant approach depicts a causal, interactive view of person–environment that separates disease from health. A few recent investigators present a more holistic description of the personal meaning of the total health experience.

WELLNESS-ILLNESS CONTINUUM

Concepts in this section include well-being, quality of life (incorporating life satisfaction), adaptation, and functional ability. However, studies selected for their relevance to one concept, for example, adaptation, often include as outcome variables other concepts of health such as well-being and life satisfaction. The categories, therefore, are not mutually exclusive.

Well-being

A sense of well-being has been identified as an important factor in health. Reed (1987) examined spirituality and well-being in a descriptive study of three groups of adults ($r = 100$ each) designed to control for terminal illness and hospitalization. Data were based on the Spiritual Perspective Scale formerly developed by the author as a test of religious perspective (Reed, 1986a) and the Index of Well-Being constructed by Campbell, Converse, and Rodgers (1976). Well-being was high in all groups, whereas perceived health was rated lowest in the terminally ill group. Planned comparisons of analysis of variance indicated that the terminally ill hospitalized patients had a greater spiritual perspective than either nonterminally ill hospitalized patients or healthy nonhospitalized persons ($p = .02$). These findings indicated the coexistence of well-being with "poor" health and suggest the fallacy of the wellness–illness dichotomy. One wonders if it will be possible one day to refer to people as the terminally healthy? The generally high scores on well-being in all groups, however, leads one to question the findings on the basis of a social desirability factor in the Index of Well-Being.

Fehring, Brennan, and Keller (1987) examined psychological and spiritual well-being in two groups ($n_1 = 95$, $n_2 = 75$) of college students with the intent of identifying spiritual well-being as a mediating factor in depression. Variables were measured by the Spiritual Well-Being scale (Paloutzian & Ellison, 1982), Kauffman's Religious Life Scale (Kauffman, 1979), and the Beck Depression Inventory (Beck & Beamesderfer, 1974). Although findings supported a negative relationship between spiritual well-being and depression, the sample was a relatively undepressed group and the relationship was mostly attributable to existential well-being and life change.

The theoretical framework for Mason's (1988) descriptive study of well-being of older women stems from a basic assumption of temporal rhythmicity in all living organisms. Mason presented literature that supported a relationship between decreased amplitude of body temperature rhythm and greater variability in the timing of the period in older adults. On that basis, she hypothesized that amplitudes of body temperature and subjective activation rhythms (measured by Hoskins' modification of Thayer's Activation–Deactivation Adjective Checklist [Hoskins, 1979; Thayer, 1967, 1978]) would be related positively to well-being (measured by a modified version of the Dupuy General Well-Being Questionnaire [Dupuy, 1973]). Also, Mason hypothesized that desynchrony of the rhythms would be negatively related to well-being. Neither hypothesis was supported. There was a suggestion in the findings that the temperature rhythm was affected by disruptive life events. However, there were distinct differences between individuals: One subject with a disturbed sleep pattern displayed no rhythmicity in his or her temperature or arousal measures, whereas another subject with disturbed sleep pattern had distinct rhythmicity in the variables measured as well as a high score on well-being. The leap between theory and operationalization may be ill-grounded, for example, human diversity/complexity was operationalized as a within-group variability rather than intraindividual variability. The connection between physiological rhythms and inner experience is reasonable from a unitary perspective but involves bridging a gap between different levels of reality. In addition, group data do not adequately capture the specifics of this connection in individual patterns over time.

Quality of Life

The definitional ambiguity of quality of life as it relates to health was the focus of several investigations. Magilvy (1985) and Burckhardt (1985) have each tested causal models to identify variables that mediate the effects of disease, disability, and other personal–environmental factors on quality of life. Social support and degree of impairment were important variables in both models. Both investigators operationalized quality of life primarily as life satisfaction.

Two independent research teams, Ferrans and Powers (1985) and Padilla and Grant (1985), have developed scales to measure quality of life, and both scales are referred to as the Quality of Life Index. Ferrans and Powers considered life satisfaction as the primary dimension of quality of life but also include an assessment of physical health and functioning, health care, and specific psychosocial factors, as well as general happiness and satisfaction. Their scale is intended for healthy populations and can be adapted for disease-related populations, as it was for dialysis patients. Evidence was presented for (a) content validity on the basis that items were supported by literature review and by reports from dialysis patients, (b) criterion-related validity by correlation with response to an overall question regarding life satisfaction ($r = 0.75$ graduate students, $r = 0.65$ dialysis patients), (c) test–retest reliability ($r = 0.87$ graduate students , $r = 0.81$ dialysis patients), and (d) internal consistency (Cronbach's alpha $= 0.93$ graduate students, and 0.90 dialysis patients).

Padilla, Grant and colleagues (Padilla & Grant, 1985; Padilla et al., 1983) developed their Quality of Life Index specifically for use with cancer patients and included the dimensions of physical function, personal attitudes and/or affective states, well-being, and support. The original 14-item scale was revised to include items for colostomy patients, resulting in a 23-item scale clustered in three groups: general physical condition, normal human activities, and personal attitudes. Factor analysis indicated that psychological well-being was the most important factor.

Quality of life is clearly a multidimensional construct with life satisfaction or psychological well-being as the primary factors. It is not clear what purpose will be served in continuing to use the summary construct.

Adaptation

Asserting that nursing's principal aim is to help people adapt, Erickson and Swain (1982) clearly endorsed the adaptive model of health. They conducted a descriptive study of hospitalized adult medical–surgical patients to determine if a person's potential to adapt to stress could be ascertained and used as a predictor of hospital stay. Several well-developed scales from the work of Gottschalk and Gleser (1969) were used to measure anxiety, hope, and feelings of tenseness, sadness, and depression. Three levels of adaptation— equilibrium (nonstress), arousal (fight–flight stress response), and impoverishment (conservative-withdrawal stress response)—were demonstrated by Mahalanobis distances between states ($p < .005$). The mean length of hospitalization for the nonstressed group was significantly less than for the combined arousal and impoverishment groups ($p = .03$). Generalization from the findings, however, is limited as the total sample was small, with only 4 and 11 subjects in the arousal and impoverished groups respectively. Replication of this study with a larger sample would have important implications for practice by helping to distinguish individuals whose adaptive potential is too low to cope with the stress of additional treatment.

Several studies focused on adaptation or adjustment to chronic illness.

Pollack (1986), in a descriptive study of adaptation to chronic illness, theorized that physiological and psychosocial adaptive responses would be related to the characteristic of hardiness, a combination of the dimensions of commitment, challenge, and belief in internal–external locus of control. The Health-Related Hardiness Scale, previously developed by the author as a modification of the Kobasa Hardiness Scale (Kobasa, 1979), was used to test three groups of adults differentiated by the diagnoses of diabetes, hypertension, and rheumatoid arthritis. Three separate tests to measure physiologic adaptation according to diagnosis were developed by the investigator and validated by a panel of experts. Only the diabetic group demonstrated a relationship between hardiness and adaptation. The selection of the sample, with 20 subjects in each of the above groups, appeared to set the stage for a comparison *between* groups. However, correlation statistics were used to relate the variables *within* each group, and the small number in each group rendered the power of the statistic quite low. Given that limitation, the effect size of the relationship within the diabetic group appeared to be strong. These results suggest that the characteristics of hardiness are adaptive for persons with diabetes but not so for persons with other disease configurations. Could this mean that the pattern of persons with diabetes is one that responds to control, whereas the patterns of persons with hypertension and arthritis are ones in which control is part of the difficulty? Further research is needed to determine the relevancy of particular coping strategies to the overall pattern of the person manifesting a particular disease.

Other studies of adjustment to chronic illness included a large study by Powers and Jalowiec (1987), in which they identified eight variables accounting for 40% of the variance in hypertension control and 19 variables accounting for 42% of the variance in adjustment to illness. However, the combination of variables identified as predictors was diverse and not easily related to each other in a meaningful way, for example, the predictors of hypertension control included both more illness-related job problems and better health adjustment scores. Dimond, McCance, and King (1987) conducted a longitudinal study of the adjustment of older adults to forced residential relocation and concluded that most older people adjust quite well. The lack of data on some subjects prior to the move and on all subjects during the initial period following the move precluded the identification of factors that facilitated their adjustment.

The adjustment patterns of chronically ill adults and their spouses (30 dyads) were the focus of an investigation by Foxall, Ekberg, and Griffith (1985). Adjustment was measured by the Life Satisfaction Index-Z Scale (Wood, Wylie, & Sheafor, 1969) and by the Older American Resource Service (OARS) Multidimensional Functional Assessment Questionnaire (Pfeiffer, 1978), and disability was rated on a 5-point scale. No significant differences were found between the ill subjects and their spouses on overall measures of these variables. Interestingly, 70% to 80% of both groups indicated that they were well satisfied with their lives and experienced congruence with their desired and achieved goals.

Sexton and Munro (1985) conducted another study of spouses' experiences of chronic illness. They compared the response of married women whose husbands had chronic obstructive pulmonary disease with married women whose husbands were without the disease on the following tests: the Subjective Stress Scale (Chapman et al., 1966), Life Satisfaction Index-A (Neugarten, Havinghurst, & Tobin, 1961), and the Illness Impact Form (Gallo, 1977). An additional 24 items developed by the investigator were added to measure the impact of the husband's illness on the wife's activities. Analysis of covariance (with age of wife and occupation of husband as covariates) revealed that women whose husbands were chronically ill reported higher levels of stress ($p = .032$) and lower life satisfaction ($p = .006$). Married women with chronically ill husbands found their usual roles in the family were expanded to include the caretaker role, increased decision-making, financial management, and day-to-day tasks. These women rated their health lower, complained of more chronic disorders, and reported less sexual activity and interest than the comparison wives. The conclusions of this study were documented carefully with statistical analyses and relationship to previous research, accentuating the importance of considering the health of the spouse as well as that of the identified patient.

Sexton and Munro (1988) extended their 1985 study by increasing the size of the sample and focusing specifically on women with and without chronic obstructive pulmonary disease (COPD). Based on t-tests of difference, women with COPD had higher levels of stress ($p = 0.003$) and lower levels of life satisfaction ($p = 0.000$) than the women without COPD. Women with COPD identified problems related to limitations imposed by the disease; yet half of this group reported their relationship with their spouse was closer than in the past. More detailed, qualitative descriptions of such relationships would be helpful in understanding this experience.

Forsyth, Delaney, and Gresham (1984) used an open-ended investigator-developed interview guide to assess the effect of chronic illness on adults' lifestyle, to identify needs arising from hospitalization and to ascertain what participants thought about health care. Through theoretical sampling to identify persons with a progressive, uncontrolled disease, 50 persons were included in the study. A constant comparative method of analysis was used to identify emerging themes and hypotheses. Interviewees emphasized their own active participation in the process of coping with chronic illness, a need to try to control the process (i.e., stay ahead of it) and maintain hope, and an intense need to be understood. This study represents a beginning contribution to the personal meaning of integrating chronic disease with subjects' self-concept, but the timing of the data collection during hospitalization tended to emphasize the break with their adjusted concepts of self and functioning, rather than the longitudinal process. The emerging theme of "winning" against the disease emphasized the subjects' concept of health as absence of disease; yet the sense of the whole person was apparent in the integrative process.

Functional Ability

In older adult populations, functional ability is often chosen as the primary measure of health. Engle (1986) proposed to test Newman's assertions of movement and time as indicators of health (Newman, 1972; 1976; 1979). Engle related walking cadence and perceived duration to be a measure of health and functional ability as measured by the Sickness Impact Profile (Gilson, Bergner, Bobbitt, & Carter, 1978). Results indicated a positive relationship ($r = .29$, $p < .01$) between walking cadence and functional ability and supported previous research findings of an inverse relationship between movement and time. The introduction of a quantitative functional measure of health, however, placed Engle's research within a linear wellness–illness continuum rather than a nonlinear perspective of the evolving pattern of the whole, the latter being the foundation of Newman's theory. The interpretation that faster movement/greater functional ability meant the individual was healthier was consistent with the continuum perspective. From the perspective of the evolving pattern of the whole, a particular movement pattern (either faster or slower) and the meaning associated with it would be indicative of the pattern of a person's health but would not identify the person as more or less healthy in a quantitative sense. Engle's findings should be interpreted in terms of this paradigm discrepancy.

To determine the adequacy of existing functional assessment instruments, Travis (1988) conducted an observational study of a random sample of 20 institutionalized, elderly psychiatric patients. A representative sample of eight observations at different times of day were made for each patient by the investigator using an unstructured format. The rating scales to which the observations (organized by Bloom's taxonomy of human behavior) were compared were the Plutchik Geriatric Rating Scale (Plutchik et al., 1970), Parachek Geriatric Behavior Rating Scale (Parachek, 1974), Geriatric Assessment Inventory (Schnelle & Traughber, 1983), Physical and Mental Impairment of Function and Evaluation Scale [(PAMIE) (Gurel, Linn & Linn, 1972)], and Multidimensional Observation Scale for Elderly Subjects [(MOSES) (Caspo & Short, 1987)]. Few mortality/survival behaviors were identified in the observational data. Information regarding the physical environment in which institutionalized individuals live was not well represented in the instruments nor was information regarding medication behavior.

Touch resistance was included in one of the instruments, MOSES, which the author considered as the most complete observer-rated functional assessment tool available.

Emphasizing the importance to nursing of understanding functional limitations and activity restrictions of clients, Goeppinger, Thomas, Charlton, and Lorig (1988), examined the psychometric properties of two recently developed self-administered measures of function for persons with arthritis: the Disability Score of the Health Assessment Questionnaire [(HAQ) (Fries, Spitz, & Young, 1982)] and the Total Health Score of the Arthritis Impact Measurement Scales [(AIMS) (Meenan, Gertman, & Mason, 1980)]. Two geographically separated but comparable samples, one from a rural area ($N = 90$) and one from an urban area ($N = 50$), were tested to obtain measures of reliability and validity. Test–retest measures yielded high overall correlations (.93 to .95 on the HAQ; .87 for AIMS). Lower correlations on the grip variable for rheumatoid arthritis group on the HAQ (.55) and on the dexterity measure in the osteoarthritis group on the AIMS (.41) could be attribtued to the nature of the disease condition. Internal consistency for the HAQ was .46 to .63 (for Pearson's r of categories with only two items) and .77 to .87 (for alpha coefficient on remaining categories). Alpha coefficients for the five AIMS functions ranged from .61 to .81. Correlation between the HAQ and the AIMS was .88. Both instruments discriminated among disease categories: In comparing arthritic subjects with diabetic subjects, 78% (HAQ) and 77% (AIMS) were correctly classified; in comparing the two types of arthritis, 80% (HAQ) and 85% (AIMS) were correctly classified. Two factors, gross motor activity and fine motor activity, accounted for 84% of the variance. In a comparison of the content of the two measures to nursing diagnosis categories (Kim, McFarland, & McLane, 1984), the authors found the HAQ more representative of nursing practice than the AIMS.

HEALTH AS A DEVELOPMENTAL PHENOMENON

Nursing research literature in the 1980s began to reflect a conceptualization of health derived from Rogers' (1970) theory of unitary person–environment development. The difficulty of maintaining a clear perspective, however, was apparent as investigators fluctuated back and forth between a wellness–illness polarization and a unidirectional developmental phenomenon.

Self-actualization

Laffrey (1985) set out to test the notion that self-actualization was an indication of a Rogerian view of the increased complexity of higher levels of development and that it would be reflected in growth motivated behavior in relation to health, rather than fear motivated behavior. She hypothesized that self-actualization would be related positively to health conception and to health behavior choice. [The health variables were measured by two author-developed instruments based on a wellness to illness continuum.] Neither hypothesis was supported. Laffrey questioned, after the fact, whether or not self-actualization is consistent with the Rogerian view of increasing complexity of person-environment interaction. The continuum of Laffrey's Health Behavior Scale, from prevention (lowest) to maintenance to promotion (highest) is consistent with the Smith continuum, but neither conceptualization may correspond to increasing complexity.

Fontes (1983), too, conceptualized health as self-actualization within the eudaimonistic model and was unable to support her hypotheses that self-actualization would be related to moderation in both cognition and interpersonal need. Fontes presented a complicated conceptualization with many hidden assumptions, and it is difficult to detect where fallacies may lie in the underlying logic and operationalization.

Expanding Consciousness

Several studies were conducted as a follow-up to Newman's early research on body movement and/or time perception within the context of health as expanding consciousness. Engle (1984) tested the relationship between personal tempo (walking cadence) and perceived duration of a 40-second interval in a sample of older women ($M = 76.5$ years) and found strong evidence ($r = -.40$, $p < .01$) for confirmation of the movement–time relationship. Thinking the theory needed an external criterion of health, Engle added a self-assessment measure of health on a linear Cantril scale from lack of health to perfect health but found no demonstrable relationship between the movement and time variables and self-assessment of health. The introduction of a linear measure of more or less health, however, shifted the conceptualization from the developmental patterning perspective initially espoused to the wellness–illness continuum; therefore lack of association with the self-assessment variable did not address the tenets of the original theory.

Nojima et al. (1987) experienced a similar dilemma in attempting to test the theory of expanding consciousness with measures of functional ability. They measured perceived duration (subjective production of a 40-second interval) as an index of consciousness (a ratio of subjective time to clock time) and compared a relatively impaired group of hospital in-patients ($n = 38$) with a comparable (by age and sex) group ($n = 23$) of university employee volunteers (unimpaired group). The impaired group scored lower on a Self-Evaluation Scale for Activities of Daily Living (adapted by Nojima et al. from the HAQ, Fries et al., 1982) than the unimpaired group and, contrary to the investigators' expectations, higher in level of consciousness than the impaired group. Their use of the chi square statistics for continuous data raises a question regarding inference from these analyses, but if the findings can be verified, they support the presence of expanded consciousness in the context of illness and disability.

In an effort to provide an explanation for conflicting results using time as an index of expanding consciousness with age, Newman and Gaudiano (1984) tested the relationship between depression (Beck Depression Inventory) and perceived duration (production of 40-second interval) in older adult women (M = 70.44 years). The results (r = 0.35, p < .002) supported their hypothesis that depression and subjective time are related negatively, a relationship that could intervene to diminish the postulated increasing subjective time with aging. This finding is limited by the fact that depression was relatively low among the group tested. Part of the problem in studies of aging and consciousness relates to the fact that the samples studied have been limited to fairly narrow age ranges and, therefore, have not possessed adequate variability to demonstrate changing consciousness with age. Retrospective cross-sectional comparisons point to increasing consciousness with age, but longitudinal studies are needed to substantiate the relationship.

Mentzer and Schorr (1986) observed that institutionalized elderly are often in situations of lack of control over their activities of daily living and postulated that perceived control (measured by Chang's Situational Control of Daily Activities) would be related to perceived duration, an index of consciousness (subjective time/clock time). A convenience sample of 40 women between 65 and 96 years of age, living in an extended care facility, was tested. Results did not support the hypothesized relationship. However, the mean index of consciousness was considerably higher than the indexes reported in previous studies (Newman, 1982). This factor plus the low power level associated with the sample size could explain the authors' inability to demonstrate the correlation between perceived duration and control.

The quantitative relational designs used to test time perception as an index of consciousness have been useful in sketching directions for future research on health as expanding consciousness but thus far have not portrayed adequately the underlying assumption of evolving pattern. Bramwell's life history method (Bramwell, 1984) holds promise of addressing this concern.

Bramwell (1984) presented life history for consideration as a qualitative method for the identification of human patterning and as a process of intervention within a framework of health as expanding consciousness. Preliminary development of a 2-phase cyclic procedure was employed with 8 persons over 60 years of age. In the first phase, participants were asked to note important events for each decade of their lives in preparation for 2 to 3 interviews in which participants shared their recollection of meaningful events in their lives. A final interview was conducted to elicit an overall response to the process and revisions if necessary. Tape recordings of the interviews were analyzed to identify patterning within the life cycle, defined as a rhythmic repetition of events. Bramwell does not specify the process of pattern identification, but found that the life history process provided the opportunity for participants to obtain a global perspective of themselves, a process that led to integration and heightened self-awareness. The experience of the life history process also became a starting point for further creativity. The homogeneity and size of the sample in this study limit generalization of the findings regarding the emerging themes.

Although bereavement studies were included in a previous review, Cowles' (1988) descriptive study of the survivors of murder victims is included here because of its relevance to personal expansion. Cowles conducted three in-depth interviews at 1-month intervals of 14 subjects, identified by newspaper reports or referred by participants in the study. The investigator gave a clear description of the process of data collection and analysis. The themes and patterns derived from the synthesis of the data focused on personal world expansion as the key concept. Cowles reported that during the first 4 months following the murder the survivor is subjected to intense expansion of their personal world in the form of (a) physical world expansion, new environments and unfamiliar others because of their situation as survivor of the murder victim; (b) cognitive personal world expansion, primarily searching for the meaning of the murder; (c) emotional personal world expansion, intense, diverse emotional response to their loss and the expanded physical world, often disorganized; (d) expansion into the victim's personal world, assuming responsibility to protect the victim's rights and reputation. The expansion of the person's personal world depicted in Cowles' study, when viewed from the standpoint of Prigogine's theory of dissipative structures (Prigogine, 1976), is an example of the transformation that takes place at times when the fluctuations of the maintenance functions of life are disrupted by chance events. It is a time when the system is forced to shift to a more complex level of organization and an opportunity for creative restructuring.

Personal Transformation

Reed's findings that increased spirituality and high well-being are characteristic of persons who are dying (Reed, 1986a, 1987) contributed to her view of dying as a transformative phase of adult development. Reed (1986b) examined depression in the elderly in relation to developmental resources, defined as characteristics of older adults such as the ability to transcend limitations of the present situation, to share one's wisdom, to accept one's past–present–future, and to achieve a sense of physical integrity. Using an instrument developed by the author (Developmental Resources of Later Adulthood Scale), Reed compared a group of older adults who were depressed in-patients to a group of adults considered healthy. The Center for Epidemiological Studies—Depression Scale (Radloff, 1977) was used to identify group membership. Three interviews were conducted with each subject at 6-week intervals, with all subjects in the depressed group having been discharged from the hospital at the time of the second and third interviews. A 2×3 factorial analysis of variance indicated that developmental resources were significantly lower in the depressed group across the three testing points ($p < .001$). Cross-lagged correlation suggested that in the healthy group developmental resources affect the level of depression, whereas in the depressed group, the direction of causation is the reverse.

The general conceptualization of the previous study implies a dichotomy between depression and health despite Reed's stated position to the contrary. She has suggested that *health* events such as disease, depression, and bereavement may be useful indicators of developmental change and that well-being is related less to medically defined health status than to ability to engage in activities that give life meaning, such as movement and interaction (Reed, 1986a).

Transcending options was the core variable identified in Duffy's (1984) grounded theory approach to the study of single-parent families' health promotion and disease prevention behaviors. Theoretical sampling yielded a sample of 59 subjects. Results indicated that transcending options was considered essential to the practice of health promoting and disease preventing behaviors. The concept of transcending options was defined as the high-level wellness end of the wellness–illness continuum, with seeking options and choosing options identified in descending order. These options were viewed as a cumulative developmental process: Choosing options as making selections from a perceived set of restricted choices; then seeking options as the process of redefining one's role, risking new behaviors and reaching of the family beyond their secure environment. Transcending options were seen as the integration of new behaviors and being in control of one's life.

Duffy's conceptualization could be viewed also from the standpoint of Prigogine's theory of dissipative structures (Prigogine, 1976), that is, moving from the maintenance type fluctuations of choosing options through the increasing fluctuations of selecting new options to the point of the giant fluctuation that propels the system to a new order, transcending options. Duffy provides an excellent description of the process of theoretical sampling used in this study and the content analysis that led to a testable hypothesis. A longitudinal study is needed to substantiate the theorized individual development.

DIRECTIONS FOR FUTURE STUDY

The predominant criterion of health emerging from this review is a person's ability to interact with and function in a changing environment. Health is viewed as a personal process characterized by meaning, pattern, and continuing development throughout the life process. The major difference in the conceptualizations of health lies in whether the process is viewed in a polarized, quantitative way, moving back and forth between higher and lower levels of wellness and illness, or as a unidirectional, unitary process of development.

The research findings emanating from both paradigms reveal the human being's power to transcend the limitations of disease, disability, and death. Life satisfaction and sense of well-being were used as indicators of health and were more important than physical ability but may not be essential to health. Increasingly disease and disability, and the problems associated with them, have been described as opportunities for personal transformation, which shifts the way the experience is viewed.

The different paradigms of health in nursing research are not about different phenomena, or events, but about the same phenomena viewed differently. That explains the confusion that often arises when attempting to categorize research as belonging to a particular paradigm. The research may have been conceptualized in one paradigm and operationalized in another, or the findings may demand a paradigm shift. Investigators and consumers of nursing research need to be aware of the differences in meaning imposed by these shifts, and future investigators need to clarify the implications of their own paradigmatic positions for the design and interpretation of their research.

The most compelling task for future research on health is the continuing development and refinement of methods consistent with the basic assumptions of these conceptualizations. For example, if health is an individual, personal process, then longitudinal studies that depict individual pattern development over the life span are needed. The particular constellation of factors that make up individual patterns of interaction with the environment must be described as a basis for comparison of the similarities and differences among patterns. The number of experiential studies in this review is insufficient to declare a trend in this direction, but these efforts to explore the personal meaning and pattern of disease and other disruptive events represent an important area for future research.

REFERENCES

Allen, D. G. (1987). Health, objectification, and alienation: Critical social theory and the process of defining and attaining health. In M. E. Duffy & N. J. Pender (Eds.), *Conceptual issues in health promotion* (pp. 128–137). Indianapolis: Sigma Theta Tau.

Beck, A. T., & Beamesderfer, A. (1974). Assessment of depression: The depression inventory. *Psychological Measurements in Psychopharmocology, 7*, 151–169.

Bloom M. (1975). Evaluation instruments: Tests and measurements in long-time care. In S. Sherwood (Ed.), *Long-term care: A handbook for researchers, planners, and providers* (573–638). New York: Spectrum Publishers.

Bramwell, L. (1984). Use of the life history in pattern identification and health promotion. *Advances in Nursing Science, 7*(1), 37–44.

Burckhardt, C. S. (1985). The impact of arthritis on quality of life. *Nursing Research, 34*, 11–18.

Campbell, A., Converse, P. E., & Rodgers, W. L. (1976). *The quality of American life: Perceptions, evaluations and satisfactions.* New York: Russell Sage Foundation.

Campbell, J. (1980). The relationship of nursing and self-awareness. *Advances in Nursing Science, 2*(4), 15–26.

Chapman, J. M., Reeder, L. G., Massey, F. J., Borun, E. R., Picken, B., Browning, C. G., Coulson, A. H., & Zimmerman, D. H. (1966). Relationship of stress, tranquilizers and serum cholesterol levels in a sample population under study for coronary heart disease. *American Journal of Epidemiology, 83*, 537–547.

Cowles, K. V. (1988). Personal world expansion for survivors of murder victims. *Western Journal of Nursing Research, 10*, 687–698.

Cox, C. L. (1987). Assumptions and challenges inherent in the conceptual dilemmas of health and health promotion. In M. E. Duffy & N. J. Pender (Eds.), *Conceptual issues in health promotion* (pp. 24–28). Indianapolis: Sigma Theta Tau.

Crawford, G. (1982). The concept of pattern in nursing: Conceptual development and measurement. *Advances in Nursing Science, 5*(1), 1–6.

Dimond, M., McCance, K., & King, K. (1987). Forced residential relocation: Its impact on the well-being of older adults. *Western Journal of Nursing Research, 9*, 445–460.

Duffy, M. (1984). Transcending options: Creating a milieu for practicing high level wellness. *Health Care for Women International, 5*, 145–161.

Dupuy, H. J. (1973). The psychological section of the current health and nutrition examination survey. *Proceedings of the Public Health Conference on Records and Statistics, Meeting Jointly with the National Conference on Mental Health Statistics, 14th National Meeting June 12–15, 1972.* Washington, DC: U.S. Government Printing Office.

Engle, V. (1984). Newman's conceptual framework and the measurement of older adults' health. *Advances in Nursing Science, 7*(1), 24–36.

Engle, V. F. (1986). The relationship of movement and time to older adults' functional health. *Research in Nursing & Health, 9*, 123–130.

Erickson, H., & Swain, M. A. (1982). A model for assessing potential adaptation to stress. *Research in Nursing & Health, 5*, 93–102.

Evans, S. K. (1979). Descriptive criteria for the concept of depleted health potential. *Advances in Nursing Science, 1*(1), 67–74.

Fehring, R. J., Brennan, P. F., & Keller, M. L. (1987). Psychological and spiritual well-being in college students. *Research in Nursing & Health, 10,* 391–398.

Ferrans, C. E., & Powers, M. J. (1985). Quality of life index: Development and psychometric properties. *Advances in Nursing Science, 8*(1), 15–24.

Fitzpatrick, J. J. (1983). A life perspective rhythm model. In J. J. Fitzpatrick & A. L. Whall (Eds.), *Conceptual models of nursing: Analysis and application* (pp. 295–302). Bowie, MD: Brady.

Fontes, H. M. (1983). An exploration of the relationships between cognitive style, interpersonal needs, and the eudiamonistic model of health. *Nursing Research, 32,* 92–96.

Forsyth, G. L., Delaney, K. D., & Gresham, M. L. (1984). Vying for a winning position: Management style of the chronically ill. *Research in Nursing & Health, 7,* 181–188.

Foxall, M. J., Ekberg, J. Y., & Griffith, N. (1985). Adjustment patterns of chronically ill middle aged persons and spouses. *Western Journal of Nursing Research, 7,* 425–441.

Fries, J. F., Spitz, P. W., & Young, D. Y. (1982). The dimensions of health outcomes: The Health Assessment Questionnaire, disability and pain scales. *The Journal of Rheumatology, 9,* 789–793.

Gallo, B. M. (1977). Home care project for COPD patients. Unpublished manuscript, Visiting Nurses Association of Hartford, Inc. Hartford, CT: Visiting Nurses Association of Hartford, Inc.

Gilson, B., Bergner, M. Bobbitt, R., & Carter, W. (1978). *The SIP: Final development and testing, 1975–1978.* Seattle: Department of Health and Community Medicine, University of Washington.

Goeppinger, J., Thomas, M. A., Charlton, S. L., & Lorig, K. (1988). A nursing perspective on the assessment of function in persons with arthritis. *Research in Nursing & Health, 11,* 321–332.

Gottschalk, L. A., & Gleser, G. C. (1969). *The measurement of psychological states through the content analysis of verbal behavior.* Berkeley: University of California Press.

Gurel, L., Linn, M. W., & Linn, B. S. (1972). Physical and mental impairment of function evaluation in the aged: The PAMIE scale. *Journal of Gerontology, 27,* 83–90.

Hall, B. A. (1981). The change paradigm in nursing: Growth versus persistence. *Advances in Nursing Science, 3*(4), 1–6.

Helmes, E., Caspo, K. G., & Short, J. A. (1987). Standardization and validation of the multidimensional observation scale for elderly subjects (MOSES). *Journal of Gerontology, 42,* 395–405.

Hollen, P. (1981). A holistic model of individual and family health based on a continuum of choice. *Advances in Nursing Science, 3*(4), 27–42.

Hoskins, C. (1979). Level of activation, body temperature, and interpersonal conflict in family relationships. *Nursing Research, 28,* 154–160.

Johnson, D. E. (1980). The behavioral system model for nursing. In J. P. Riehl & C. Roy (Eds.), *Conceptual models for nursing practice* (2nd ed.) (pp. 207–216). New York: Appleton-Century-Crofts.

Kauffman, J. H. (1979). Social correlates of spiritual maturity among North American mennonites. In D. Moberg (Ed.), *Spiritual well-being: Sociological perspectives* (pp. 237–254). Washington, DC: University Press of America.

Keller, M. J. (1981). Toward a definition of health. *Advances in Nursing Science, 4*(1), 43–64.

Kim, M. J., McFarland, G. K., & McLane, A. M. (Eds.) (1984). *Pocket guide to nursing diagnosis*. St. Louis: Mosby.

Kobasa, S. C. (1979). Stressful life events, personality, and health: An inquiry into hardiness. *Journal of Personality and Social Psychology, 37*(1), 1–11.

Laffrey, S. C. (1985). Health behavior choice as related to self-actualization and health conception. *Western Journal of Nursing Research, 7,* 279–294.

Laffrey, S. C. (1986). Development of a health conception scale. *Research in Nursing & Health, 9,* 107–114.

Laffrey, S. C., Loveland-Cherry, C. J., & Winkler, S. J. (1986). Health behavior: Evolution of two paradigms. *Public Health Nursing, 3,* 92–100.

Magilvy, J. K. (1985). Quality of life of hearing-impaired older women. *Nursing Research, 34,* 140–144.

Mason, D. J. (1988). Circadian rhythms of temperature and activation and the well-being of older women. *Nursing Research, 37,* 276–281.

Meenan, R. F., Gertman, P. M., & Mason, J. H. (1980). Measuring health status in arthritis: The Arthritis Impact Measurement Scales. *Arthritis and Rheumatism, 23,* 146–151.

Mentzer, C. A., & Schorr, J. A. (1986). Perceived situational control and perceived duration of time: expressions of life patterns. *Advances in Nursing Science, 9*(1), 12–20.

Miller, E. R., & Parachek, J. F. (1974). Validation and standardization of a goal-oriented, quick-screening geriatric scale. *Journal of the American Geriatrics Society, 22,* 278–283.

Muhlenkamp, A. F. (1987). Health as an individual phenomenon: Investigative dilemmas. In M. E. Duffy & N. J. Pender (Eds.), *Conceptual issues in health promotion* (pp. 82–90). Indianapolis: Sigma Theta Tau.

Narayan, S. M., & Joslin, D. J. (1980). Crisis theory and intervention: A critique of the medical model and proposal of a holistic nursing model. *Advances in Nursing Science, 2*(4), 27–40.

Neugarten, B., Havinghurst, R., & Tobin, S. (1961). The measurement of life satisfaction. *Journal of Gerontology, 16,* 134–143.

Newman, M. A. (1972). Time estimation in relation to gait tempo. *Perceptual and Motor Skills, 34,* 359–366.

Newman, M. A. (1976). Movement tempo and the experience of time. *Nursing Research, 25,* 273–279.

Newman, M. A. (1979). *Theory development in nursing*. Philadelphia: Davis.

Newman, M. A. (1982). Time as an index of expanding consciousness with age. *Nursing Research, 31,* 290–293.

Newman, M. A. (1983). Newman's health theory. In I. Clements & F. Roberts (Eds.), *Family health: A theoretical approach to nursing care* (pp. 161–175). New York: Wiley.

Newman, M. A. (1986). *Health as expanding consciousness*. St. Louis: Mosby.

Newman, M. A. (1987). Patterning. In M. E. Duffy & N. J. Pender (Eds.), *Conceptual issues in health promotion* (pp. 36–50). Indianapolis: Sigma Theta Tau.

Newman, M., & Gaudiano, J. (1984). Depression as an explanation for decreased subjective time in the elderly. *Nursing Research, 33,* 137–139.

Nojima, Y., Oda, A., Nishii, H., Fukui, M., Seo, K., & Akiyoshi, H. (1987). Perception of time among Japanese inpatients. *Western Journal of Nursing Research, 9,* 288–298.

Norbeck, J. S. (1987). Empiricism and health promotion research. In M. E. Duffy &

N. J. Pender (Eds.), *Conceptual issues in health promotion* (pp. 110–120). Indianapolis: Sigma Theta Tau.

Padilla, G. V., & Grant, M. M. (1985). Quality of life as a cancer nursing outcome variable. *Advances in Nursing Science, 8*(1), 45–60.

Padilla, G. V., Presant, C., Grant, M. M., Metter, G., Lipsett, J., & Heide, F. (1983). Quality of life index for patients with cancer. *Research in Nursing & Health, 6,* 117–126.

Paloutzian, R., & Ellison, C. (1982). Loneliness, spiritual well-being and quality of life. In L. Peplau & D. Perlman (Eds.), *Loneliness: A sourcebook of current theory, research and therapy* (pp. 224–237). New York: Wiley.

Parse, R. R. (1981). *Man-living-health: A theory of nursing.* New York: Wiley.

Parse, R. R. (1987). *Nursing science: Major paradigms, theories, and critiques.* Philadelphia: Saunders.

Pender, N. J. (1984). Health promotion and illness prevention. In H. H. Werley & J. J. Fitzpatrick (Eds.), *Annual review of nursing research, Vol. 3* (pp. 83–106). New York: Springer Publishing Co.

Pender, N. J. (1987). Health and health promotion: The conceptual dilemmas. In M. E. Duffy & N. J. Pender (Eds.), *Conceptual Issues in Health Promotion* (pp. 7–23). Indianapolis: Sigma Theta Tau.

Pfeiffer, E. (1978). *OARS Multidimensional Functional Assessment Questionnaire.* Durham, NC: Duke University Center for the Study of Aging and Human Development.

Plutchik, R., Conte, H., Lieberman, M., Bakur, M., Grossman, J., & Lehrman, N. (1970). Reliability and validity of a scale for assessing the functioning of geriatric patients. *Journal of the American Geriatric Society, 18,* 491–500.

Pollack, S. E. (1986). Human responses to chronic illness: Physiologic and psychologic adaptation. *Nursing Research, 35,* 90–97.

Powers, M. J., & Jalowiec, A. (1987). Profile of the well-controlled, well-adjusted hypertensive patient. *Nursing Research, 36,* 106–110.

Prigogine, I. (1976). Order through fluctuation: Self-organization and social system. In E. Jantsch & C. H. Waddington (Eds.), *Evolution and consciousness* (pp. 93–133). Reading, MA: Addison-Wesley.

Radloff, L. S. (1977). The CES-D scale: A self-report depression scale for research in the general population. *Applied Psychological Measurement, 1,* 385–401.

Reed, P. G. (1983). Implications of the life-span developmental framework for well-being in adulthood and aging. *Advances in Nursing Science, 6*(1), 18–25.

Reed, P. G. (1986a). Religiousness among terminally ill and healthy adults. *Research in Nursing & Health, 9,* 35–42.

Reed, P. G. (1986b). Developmental resources and depression in the elderly. *Nursing Research, 35,* 368–374.

Reed, P. G. (1987). Spirituality and well-being in terminally ill hospitalized adults. *Research in Nursing & Health, 10,* 335–344.

Reynolds, C. L. (1988). The measurement of health in nursing research. *Advances in Nursing Science, 10*(4), 23–31.

Rogers, M. E. (1970). *An introduction to the theoretical basis of nursing.* Philadelphia: Davis.

Roy, C. (1976). *Introduction to nursing: An adaptation model.* Englewood Cliffs, NJ: Prentice-Hall.

Schnelle, J. F., & Traughber, B. (1983). A behavioral assessment system applicable to geriatric nursing facility residents. *Behavioral Assessment, 5,* 231–243.

Schorr, J. A. (1983). Manifestations of consciousness and the developmental phenomenon of death. *Advances in Nursing Science, 6*(1), 26–35.

Sexton, D. L., & Munro, B. H. (1985). Impact of a husband's chronic illness (COPD) on the spouse's life. *Research in Nursing & Health, 8,* 83–90.

Sexton, D. L., & Munro, B. H. (1988). Living with chronic illness: The experience of women with chronic obstructive pulmonary disease (COPD). *Western Journal of Nursing Research, 10,* 26–38.

Smith, J. A. (1981). The idea of health: A philosophical inquiry. *Advances in Nursing Science, 3,* 43–50.

Stevenson, J. S. (1983). Adulthood: A promising focus for future research. In H. H. Werley & J. J. Fitzpatrick (Eds.), *Annual review of nursing research, Vol. 1* (pp. 55–74). New York: Springer Publishing Co.

Stevenson, J. S. (1987). Frameworks to consider and the challenges we face. In M. E. Duffy & N. J. Pender (Eds.), *Conceptual issues in health promotion* (pp. 98–108). Indianapolis: Sigma Theta Tau.

Thayer, R. E. (1967). Measurement of activation through self-report. *Psychological Reports, 20,* 663–678.

Thayer, R. E. (1978). Toward a psychological theory of multidimensional activation (arousal). *Motivation and Emotion, 2*(1), 1–34.

Travis, S. S. (1988). Observer-rated functional assessments for institutionalized elders. *Nursing Research, 37,* 138–143.

Tripp-Reimer, T. (1984). Reconceptualizing the construct of health: Integrating emic and etic perspectives. *Research in Nursing & Health, 7,* 101–110.

Tripp-Reimer, T. (1987). Using phenomenology in health promotion research. In M. E. Duffy & N. J. Pender (Eds.), *Conceptual issues in health promotion* (pp. 121–127). Indianapolis: Sigma Theta Tau.

Watson, J. (1985). *Nursing: Human science and human care.* Norwalk, CT: Appleton-Century-Crofts.

Wood, V., Wylie, M. L., & Sheafor, B. (1969). An analysis of a short self-report measure of life satisfaction: Correlation with rater judgments. *Journal of Gerontology, 24,* 465–469.

Woods, N. F. (1988). Women's health. In J. J. Fitzpatrick, R. L. Taunton, & J. Q. Benoliel (Eds.), *Annual review of nursing research, Vol. 6* (pp. 209–236). New York: Springer Publishing Co.

Woods, N. F., Laffrey, S., Duffy, M., Lentz, M. J., Mitchell, E. S., Taylor, D., & Cowan, K. A. (1988). Being healthy: Women's images. *Advances in Nursing Science, 11*(1), 36–46.

Index

Contents of Previous Volumes

ORDER FORM

Save 10% on Volume 10 with this coupon.

____ Check here to order the ANNUAL REVIEW OF NURSING RESEARCH, Volume 10, 1992 at a 10% discount. You will receive an invoice requesting pre-payment.

Save 10% on all future volumes with a continuation order.

____Check here to place your continuation order for the ANNUAL REVIEW OF NURSING RESEARCH. You will receive a pre-payment invoice with a 10% discount upon publication of each new volume, beginning with Volume 10, 1992. You may pay for prompt shipment or cancel with no obligation.

Name _____

Institution _____

Address _____

City/State/Zip _____

Examination copies for possible course adoption are available to instructors "on approval" only. Write on institutional letterhead, noting course, level, present text, and expected enrollment (Include $3.00 for postage and handling). Prices slightly higher overseas. Prices subject to change.

_____

Mail this coupon to:
SPRINGER PUBLISHING COMPANY
536 Broadway, New York, N.Y. 10012